Interracial Romance
and Health

I0110266

Interracial Romance and Health

Bridging Generations, Race Relations, and Well-Being

Byron Miller

LEXINGTON BOOKS
Lanham • Boulder • New York • London

Published by Lexington Books
An imprint of The Rowman & Littlefield Publishing Group, Inc.
4501 Forbes Boulevard, Suite 200, Lanham, Maryland 20706
www.rowman.com

6 Tinworth Street, London SE11 5AL, United Kingdom

Copyright © 2023 The Rowman & Littlefield Publishing Group, Inc.

All rights reserved. No part of this book may be reproduced in any form or by any electronic or mechanical means, including information storage and retrieval systems, without
written permission from the publisher, except by a reviewer who may quote passages
in a review.

British Library Cataloguing in Publication Information Available

Library of Congress Cataloging-in-Publication Data Available

ISBN 978-1-7936-3405-4 (cloth: alk. paper)
ISBN 978-1-7936-3406-1 (electronic)
ISBN 978-1-7936-3407-8 (pbk.: alk. paper)

♾™ The paper used in this publication meets the minimum requirements of American
National Standard for Information Sciences—Permanence of Paper for Printed Library
Materials, ANSI/NISO Z39.48-1992.

This book is dedicated to all the past, present, and future Bridge Kids!!

Contents

Acknowledgments

Writing this book would not have been possible without the help of many people, all of whom cannot be named, so I want to first thank anyone who has ever loved and supported me. This list begins with my mother, for showing me love on this earth, and my father, who continues to motivate me from heaven. Thanks to my siblings Gerald, Darren, Daphne, and Bobby, from whom I have learned much. I also recognize people like Uncle Mac, Grimace, and Martin, for being my role models, as well as Breigh, Brandon, Blake, Quentin, Korey, and Jayden, for pretending to let me be theirs.

I must acknowledge my inspiring upbring in Rochester, New York. Nicknamed the "World's Image City"; it is the home of Frederick Douglass, Susan B. Anthony, East High School, and where I developed my sociological imagination way before I heard the concept. So, I wouldn't have made it this far personally or professionally without my Rochester family including Adam, Chuck, Erik, Nells, and Mrs. Hunter, to name a few of many.

I acknowledge the impact Chris Ponticelli, Barbara Cruz, R. Jay Turner, and others had on my academic career. Thanks to Robin Simon for always making me excited to pursue this topic, and Verna Keith for being an inspiration and a mentor. A special acknowledgment must go to Kay Pasley, for planting the seed for me to write this book, and to my cousin Art, for encouraging me to follow through on that suggestion.

I extend much gratitude to my colleagues Cap, Roudi, Sara, and Doc for their willingness to collaborate with me on this project. An extra-big hug to you Doc, for being the friend, mentor, and colleague who has spent more than a decade helping me hone my conceptualization of the Bridge Kids. Along those lines, I want to send a big thank-you to all the students and young people who continuously motivate me to help end racism so future generations can feel free to love whomever they want to love. Go Noles! Go Bulls!

Introduction

Roudi Nazarinia Roy and Anthony G. James Jr.

An axiom common to thinking about relationships is the notion that "Love Is Blind," which suggests that love is all that is needed to develop and sustain a lasting and satisfying relationship. While this may be the case for some relationships, not all relations are created equal. In this vein, we are specifically referring to that of interracial relationships, particularly as it relates to the challenges facing couples in society. Simply put, the successful maintenance of an interracial relationships requires more than the mere love of one's partner. Beyond love, factors such as how much you are willing to sacrifice for your partner and/or how much of your privilege you are willing to give up, may be more apt questions for determining the development and maintenance of successful interracial relationships. Moreover, what interracial couples have to create is a union that supports each partner's daily encounters in a society that continues to place race, and its limited categories, at the forefront of how we judge people. That is the focus of this introductory chapter. We take a historical view to help set the stage for the content covered in the chapters that follow.

In the United States, there is an undeniable instability in interracial relationships and these numbers vary based on the racial composition of the couple, with White-Black unions having the highest rate of instability (Bratter & King, 2008). In fact, Bratter and King (2008) found not only racial differences in marital instability, but also gender differences. For example, marriages between a non-Hispanic Black male and a White woman were twice as likely to end in divorce, and Asian males married to a White woman were 59 percent more likely to experience a divorce than a marriage between a White male and a White female. Interestingly, these divorce rates were different when the gender of the Black or Asian spouse was female. Such that White men married to Black women were 44 percent less likely to divorce than a marriage between a White male and a White female. Asian women married

1

to White men were only 4 percent more likely to divorce than a White male married to a White female.

The greater levels of instability for interracial relationships are not only attributed to the internal dynamics of the couple's relationship but also caused by factors outside of their relationship, from close encounters with family (Kalmijn, Graaf & Janssen, 2005) to an overall society (Zhang & Van Hook, 2009) that disapproves of such a union. When two individuals from varying racial backgrounds enter a romantic union, each member of the couple will be challenged by other members of their own social groups. Thus, the extent to which each member of the couple is willing to sustain efforts to rebut the challenges will be important for the duration and satisfaction of the relationship. This requires members of the couple to remain open and willing to accept the realities that face their relationship. This level of commitment to one's partner, and the deeper level of understanding for one's partner (Leslie & Letiecq, 2004) given the inevitable challenges that both partners will face, creates a unique connection among individuals in interracial relationships (Roy, 2019). A connection that withstands decades of discrimination because partners are committed to each other and the family they have come together to create (Roy & Rollins, 2019). To fully understand these current-day realities, we must journey across time and explore the history of race and interracial relationships in America. Only then can we begin to fully discuss the realities of intimate relationships, parenting, and the realities of being a mixed-race family in the United States.

A HISTORY OF INTERRACIAL RELATIONSHIP

Although many, particularly interracial couples and multiracial families, now celebrate the *Loving v. Virginia* (1967) Supreme Court case that struck down state laws banning interracial marriage in the United States, it becomes easy to overlook how the very same type of interracial relationships (i.e., *Pace v. Alabama*) gave rise to the anti-miscegenation laws. Millward (2010) argues the willful ignorance of celebrating the achievement of *Loving v. Virginia* without acknowledging the fact that interracial relationships have a strong presence in American history, particularly during the era of slavery, when slave masters could engage in sexual relations with their female slaves. Millward (2010) explains that slave owners who developed emotions for the female slaves could provide a residence for them and their offspring and, in some regions of the country, also free these women with whom they had sexual relations and ultimately their offspring because slavery was inheritable. But Black women were considered property during antebellum and as such were not able to consent to any type of relationship with White slave owners or even male slaves. Put plainly, this created an unequal foundation from which these unions were birthed.

Fast-forward from the days of legalized slavery to around 1883, when a Black man (Tony Pace) engaged in sexual relations with a White woman (Mary Cox) in Alabama. The pair were subsequently arrested, each given a two-year prison sentence, and the Supreme Court sanctioned racial separation with its ruling on *Pace v. Alabama* (1883), affirming anti-miscegenation laws (Bryant & Duncan, 2019). According to Webb and colleagues (2019), this ruling gave states the authority to pass racially restrictive laws like Virginia's Racial Integrity Act of 1924 requiring race to be identified on birth records, manufacturing the "one drop rule" *rule* of labeling people with any African ancestry as Black (Jordan, 2014; Wolfe, 2015) as an attempt to keep the White bloodline pure. These laws serve as the root cause for challenges of interracial relationships in the United States and created a strong social stigma and negative perceptions of such unions. Further, these laws helped entrench desires to segregate racial groups, which eventually allowed anti-miscegenation laws to reach the federal level in the Loving case.

The passing of the *Loving v. Virginia* (1967) ruling did not, however, remove all types of discrimination against interracial relationships as Southern states were slow to acknowledge such rulings. Five decades later, discrimination against interracial relationships and mixed-race families continues across the United States in varying degrees based on geographic locations. Over these past five decades, however, researchers have sought to answer questions such as: Who engages in interracial relationships?; How acceptable are interracial relationships?; and How stable are such relationships?

WHO ENGAGES IN INTERRACIAL RELATIONSHIPS?

For some, the increase in interracial marriages in the United States is a symbol of improving race relations (Fu & Heaton, 2008; Ono & Berg, 2010), and although it is common to use the 1967 U.S. Supreme Court ruling in *Loving v. Virginia* as the birth of such unions, interracial marriages took place well before the passing of this law. In fact, Ono and Berg (2010) document the increase in Japanese and Japanese American marriages to White Americans during World War II, decades *before* the *Loving v. Virginia* ruling, as an indication of improving race relations between the two groups. The anti-miscegenation laws were mainly used to prevent Black and White marriages (Zhang & Van Hook, 2009), and thus we see after the *Loving v. Virginia* 1967 ruling, a steady increase in Black and White marriages in the United States. Furthermore, states had varying anti-miscegenation laws that contributed to distinct differences in opportunities and privileges across groups such that marriages between White and Asians were allowed, while anti-miscegenation laws prohibited the same rights to Black Americans' and American Indians' unions (Bialik, 2017).

For example, in 1967 when the *Loving v. Virginia* ruling was passed, 3 percent of newlyweds were married to someone of another race or ethnicity (Bialik, 2017). In 1970, all marriages between spouses of different races, including White, Black, Asian, and American Indian, was at 1 percent (Wang, 2012), rose to 3 percent by the late 1970s and early 1980s (Bialik, 2017), and to more than 5 percent in 2000 (Zhang & Van Hook, 2009). From 1980 to 2008, there was a steady increase in interracial marriages between Black and White Americans but a delayed increase in marriages between other minority groups and White Americans (Qian & Lichter, 2011). Based on data from the 1980 US Census and the 2008 American Community Survey, Qian and Lichter (2011) suggest that the increase in Asian and Latin American immigrants has resulted in fewer interracial and interethnic marriages between White American and Asian or Latino Americans. This would suggest that the increase in interracial unions has not only occurred in net numbers, but also in the diversity of those unions.

In 2013, 6.3 percent of all marriages were between spouses of different races (Wang, 2012). More specifically, 12 percent of newlyweds were in interracial marriages (7 percent White, 19 percent Black, 28 percent Asian, and 58 percent American Indian), not considering interracial marriage between Hispanic and non-Hispanic individuals (Wang, 2012). There are also distinct gender gaps between interracial marriages amongst Black men (25 percent) and Black women (12 percent) marrying outside their race. The opposite trend occurred among Asian Americans, with a greater percentage of Asian women (37 percent) marrying outside their race than Asian men (16 percent) (Wang, 2012). The distribution of interracial marriages across the sexes among White Americans and American Indians were relatively similar.

In addition to greater immigration, it has been noted that socioeconomic selectivity plays a large role in interracial coupling such that minority members in interracial relationships tend to have higher levels of socioeconomic status relative to others within their racial category (Lee & Edmonston, 2005; Wang, 2012). Accordingly, the numerous factors associated with the immigration and social mobility of racial and ethnic minorities have greatly increased their opportunities to form interracial relationships. These trends may also demonstrate that race relations and subsequent interracial unions may continue to proliferate more in some geographic regions than others, despite the strong social stigma of some stemming from a legacy of slavery and racism.

SOCIETAL VIEWS ON INTERRACIAL RELATIONSHIPS

Recall that in 1967, only 3 percent of newlyweds married someone of a different race, but in 2017, interracial marriages accounted for 17 percent of all newlyweds (Livingston & Brown, 2017). The increasing rates for interracial marriages are undoubtedly due to growing acceptance of such relationships, but as the number of interracial relationships increases, so, too, does the acceptance of them. For instance, in 1990, over 60 percent of Nonblack American adults surveyed said they would be very or somewhat opposed to a close relative marrying a Black person, but almost three decades later, that percentage has dropped to under 15 percent (Pew Research Center, 2017). In 2000, almost a quarter of Americans polled (24 percent) said interracial marriages would be good for society; just a mere four years later, this number rose to 37 percent (Pew Research Center, 2017). Negative social views of interracial marriage shifted in the opposite direction from 13 percent in 2000 to 9 percent in 2014, while the majority of those polled felt it did not make a difference for society either way (61 percent in 2000 and 52 percent in 2014).

In 2017, the level of acceptance for interracial marriages continued to grow as nearly 40 percent of American adults felt marrying someone of a different race was good for society (Livingston & Brown, 2017). Of course, these attitudes vary across demographics as people with a college degree, males, White Americans, and those living in urban communities are more likely to see marriage with someone outside of one's own race as good for society. Interestingly when asked about intermarriage in their own families, 31 percent said they would oppose such relationships in their families in 2000, but that number dropped to 9 percent in 2002, only to increase to 16 percent in 2008 (Pew Research Center, 2017), when the United States elected its first Black American president, Barack Obama.

HOW STABLE ARE INTERRACIAL RELATIONSHIPS?

The literature on the stability of interracial relationships is mixed with earlier studies on this phenomenon reporting low levels of stability among interracial couples (Batson, Qian, & Lichter, 2006; Bramlett & Mosher, 2002; Bratter & King, 2008; Crester & Leon, 1982; Fu & Wolfinger, 2011; Wang, Kao, & Joyner, 2006). In other words, these studies find that individuals in interracial marriages are more likely to divorce than those in same-race marriages. Others who compare interracial relationship to homogenous Black unions report they are relatively stable (Troy, Lewis-Smith, & Laurenceau, 2006), while other studies have demonstrated that the instability of interracial marriages are not much different than those of their homogenous counterparts (Zhang & Van Hook, 2014). For example, Black-White couples have similar stability as Black-Black couples, and Hispanic-White couples are similar to Hispanic-Hispanic couples, but Black-White *and* Hispanic-White couples both have *higher* levels of instability than White-White couples. Interestingly, Zhang and Van Hook (2014) found that interracial marriages between Asian/ White partners were more stable than White/White marriages but less stable than Asian/Asian marriages.

According to a review of the literature on marital quality and stability in interracial relationships by Bryant and Duncan (2019), not only are their differences across racial pairings, but a race by gender interaction (i.e., race*gender) of interracial couples is an important factor that must be considered. For example, White female–Black male and White female–Asian male couples were more likely to divorce than White-White couples (Bratter & King, 2008). Studies also find that Black men married to White women, Latino men married to Black women (Jones, 2010), and Latino men married to White women (Fu & Wolfinger, 2011) each have significantly higher risks of divorce. Interestingly, Bratter and King (2008) report that relationships in which the husband is of mixed Black-White ancestry are least likely to dissolve. Still others have argued that the instability in interracial relationship is due to factors already associated with a higher risk of divorce, such as lower age at marriage and multiple-partner fertility (Lichter, Quin, & Mellott, 2006; Lundquist, 2006). Regardless of the argument there is no doubt that the race of a spouse is a factor in their risk of marital dissolution.

The variations across different race pairings indicate that not all Nonwhite-White unions are equal, and Black partners continue to face greater risk factors. Some researchers have suggested that Black-White unions consistently show higher risk for instability, and they assume that structural and institutional racism against Black Americans are an important factor in their relationship instability and must not be overlooked, particularly among Black men (Jones, 2010; Zhang & Van Hook, 2014). As these couples are crossing a line that has a strong history of rejection in American (Billingsley, 1968; Miller, 2020), not surprisingly they face social discrimination that is particularly harsh (Yancey, 2007).

CHALLENGES

In many relationships the basic assumptions are that if a couple has similar characteristics, they will have greater understanding, experience less conflict, and find greater enjoyment in participating in common activities and support with family and friends (Kalmijn, 1998). When two people from different cultures come together in a relationship, it is thus expected that they will face some challenges as their differences may create greater likelihood of disagreement and misunderstandings and ultimately stress. Among interracial couples, these stressors arise from within the couple's relationship and outside of it (Roy, 2019). For example, an interracial couple may have differing perceptions of an experience such that one partner sees the interaction as racist while the other partner brushes it off as a coincidence. These experiences can take a toll on a partnership especially if they are not addressed by the couple. One partner can be left feeling as though their experience is irrelevant or that their partner cannot fully understand what it means to be of a certain race in this country.

Interracial couples also face a unique set of challenges related to familial acceptance of their relationship. Due to the currently heightened racial climate in the United States, parents in interracial relationships may seek to protect their children from involvement in a relationship that might create unwarranted stressors based on their partners racial category (Roy, 2019). The unknown and unfamiliar sometimes breeds ignorance, and some parents are unwilling to open their hearts and their minds to a potential son-in-law or daughter-in-law who is of a different race or culture. This lack of acceptance and support can be difficult and strenuous, particularly on younger adults, even if they have had a good relationship with their parents prior to their interracial relationship. But parents are not the only source of disapproval; siblings, extended family, and friends can also demonstrate disapproval of an interracial relationship that can produce equal amounts of stress.

Interestingly, we see these types of race related family dynamics play out in pop-culture films such as, *The Week Of* (2018), *A United Kingdom* (2016), *Our Family Wedding* (2010), *Fools Rush In* (1997), and *The Joy Luck Club* (1993), where families tackle issues related to interracial relationships. In addition to the challenges faced by the interracial couples in these films, we see these characters at some point also depict a strong sense of connection, understanding, and a desire to protect one another. Although interracial partners have been found to possess a heightened sensitivity for threats from outside their relationship (Henderson, 2000), they have also shown a greater level of understanding for their partner (Leslie & Letiecq, 2004). According to Leslie and Letiecq (2004), partners in interracial marriages have a heightened sense of awareness of their own racial identity as well as that of their partner, and as such, they are active in their responses to the outside world while staying focused on addressing the needs that occur in their relationship. But this strong sense of connection can be difficult to establish and maintain.

Undeniably a major challenge for interracial couples is the willingness to fight against negativity external to the relationship, which impacts internal dynamics within the union. At the core of the instability prevalent in interracial relationships are the messages and behaviors encountered through interactions with external entities. If not, this can seep into the union itself and corrode the fibers that hold it together. For example, a White woman may be called racist by her own Hispanic male partner because of a comment she made in response to one of his experiences. While frustrations are understandable, members of such relationship structures must fight vigorously to protect the fibers and foundations of their unisons. One such approach to helping with this, particularly from a social stigma perspective, is the growth of children produced in such unions. Because these unions produce children who are likely to lack such negative beliefs about mixed-race families, it can lessen the social stigma toward them as increasing numbers of them are in the population over time.

THE PROMISE OF BRIDGE KIDS

For many couples in interracial relationships, it can be a daily battle to push back against society in terms of how they view their relationship or how they view their partner. To have a partner respond in an unsupportive way, on top of that battle, can be destructive for the relationship. Members of these couples must commit to a goal of building a foundation of love, trust, and collaboration that helps create a relational mechanism that helps rebut the negativity the relationship is likely to encounter. One factor that may help partners in such practices is the desire to create a loving environment for their children. Wanting to create a loving and stable environment for children can be an incentive for coming to support one another. Further, the success of such unions can also corrode away the misbelief of them being inherently bad.

As more individuals enter interracial unions, such unions become normalized in U.S. society. Multiracial families seeking familiarity in experience, who were isolated only a few decades ago, are now seeing greater representation, in the media and in their communities (Roy & Rollins, 2019). These representations not only provide an opportunity for reflections and validation of experiences but provide those from outside these families an opportunity to see the diversity that exists within multiracial families. It is not uncommon to see mixed race families acknowledging one another in public, thereby affirming their existence. Even parents who do not initially support the interracial union tend to have a change of heart once grandchildren are born (Kang Fu, 2008; Kibria, 2002; Roy, 2019). Grandparents also have an endless love for their grandchildren with some feeling a need to reach out and make these connections, acknowledge they have a Multiracial grandchild, and even pulling out a photo and share the beauty in their grandchild. Perhaps sadly but undeniable, these grandparents join in the everlasting struggle to ensure their grandchildren do not inherit a world filled with discrimination and hate based on race.

The period of history in which individuals develop has strong impact on their conceptualizations of family and their behaviors in them (James, 2020). With *Loving v. Virginia* (1967) only being five decades old, may individuals alive today developed in environments where interracial unions were illegal. As time passes, and more individuals enter in interracial unions and start families, there will be more opportunities for those individuals to become less opposed to such unions. Similarly, as members of older generations die off, many of the negative beliefs they have about interracial relationships are likely to die with them. Lastly, the children produced in such unions are less likely to have negative views of such unions, even if only for the mere fact that they are the product of them.

Regardless of how one's family or society perceives interracial and inter-ethnic relationships these unions have and will continue to evolve over time. In particular, young adults ages eighteen to twenty-nine are most likely to approve of interracial marriage (Newport, 2013), most likely to be fine with a family member being interracially married (Passel, Wang, & Taylor, 2010), most likely to believe interracial marriage is good for society (Livingston & Brown, 2017), and most likely to engage in interracial relationships (Jones, 2005). Such attitudes and behaviors clearly suggest young adults are the most willing to "bridge" racial groups by accepting the decisions of those that cross racial lines for romance as well as becoming interracially involved themselves. Moreover, in many cases, interracial relationships will also produce multiracial children. For example, in 2017, 14 percent of newborns in the United States were identified as multiracial or multiethnic (Bialik, 2017). As with children from other family structures, these children need loving and supportive environments in order to thrive (James, Bush, & Peterson, 2016; James & Fine, 2014). With the aforementioned challenges in mind, more scholarly focus is needed that examines the impact society has on the social relationships and well-being of these "Bridge Kids," to better assess how race relations have progressed, predict where they are heading, as well as promote a functional and supportive environment that protects them against external challenges related to their interracial relationship.

REFERENCES

Batson, C. D., Qian, Z., & Lichter, D. T. (2006). Interracial and intraracial patterns of mate selection among America's diverse Black populations. *Journal of Marriage and Family, 68*(3), 658–72.

Billingsley, A. *Black families in White America*. Prentice-Hall; Englewood Cliffs, NJ: 1968.

Bialik, K. (2017). Key facts about race and marriage, 50 years after *Loving v. Virginia*, *Pew Research Center.* Retrieved from Key facts about race and marriage, 50 years after Loving v. Virginia, Pew Research Center.

Bramlett, M. D., & Mosher, W. D. (2002). Cohabitation, marriage, divorce, and remarriage in the United States. *Vital Health Statistics, 23*(22), 1–32.

Bratter, J. L., & King, R. (2008). "But will it last?": Marital instability among interracial and same-race couples. *Family Relations, 57*(2), 160–71

Bryant, C. M. & Duncan, J. C. (2019). Interracial Marriages: Historical and Contemporary Trends. In R. N. Roy & A. Rollins, (2019). *Biracial Families: Crossing Boundaries, Blending Cultures, and Challenging Racial Ideologies*. (pp. 81–104). New York, NY: Springer.

Crester, G. A., & Leon, J. J. (1982). Intermarriage in the US: An overview of theory and research. *Marriage and Family Review, 5*(1), 3–15.

Fu, X., & Heaton, T.B. (2008). Racial and educational homogamy: 1980 to 2000. *Sociological Perspectives, 51*, 735–58.

Fu, V. K., & Wolfinger, N.H. (2011). Broken boundaries or broken marriages? Racial intermarriage and divorce in the United States. *Social Science Quarterly, 92*(4), 1096–117.

Henderson, D. A. (2000). Racial/Ethnic intermarried couples and marital interaction: Marital issues and problem solving. *Sociological Focus, 33*(4), 421–38.

James, A.G., Bush, K.R., & Peterson, G., (2016). Children and youth in Stepfamilies. In T. G. and M. Bloom (Eds.), *Handbook of Childhood Behavioral Issues: Evidence-based Approaches to Prevention and Treatment* (pp. 118–36). New York: Routledge.

James, A., & Fine, M. A. (2014). Healthy Development in Children of Divorced Parents. In T. G. and M. Bloom (Eds.), *Encyclopedia of Primary Prevention and Health Promotion II* (pp. 684–91). New York: Springer Publishing Company

James, A. G. (2020) *Black Families: A Systems approach*. San Diego, CA: Cognella Press.

Jones, A. (2010). Stability of Men's Interracial First Unions: A Test of Educational Differentials and Cohabitation History. *Journal of Family and Economic Issues, 31*, 241–56

Jones, J. M. (2005). Most Americans approve of interracial dating. *Gallup*. Retrieved from http://www.gallup.com/poll/19033/Most-Americans-Approve -Interracial-Dating.aspx.

Jordan, W. D. (2014). Historical Origins of the One-Drop Racial Rule in the United States. *Journal of Critical Mixed Race Studies, 1*(1), 98–132.

Kalmijn, M. (1993). Trends in Black/White intermarriage. *Social Forces, 72*(1), 119–46.

Kalmijn, M. (1998). Intermarriage and Homogamy: Causes, Patterns, Trends. *Annual Review of Sociology, 24*, 395–421.

Kalmijn, M., De Graaf, P., & Janssen, J. (2005). Intermarriage and the risk of divorce in the Netherlands: The effects of differences in religion and in nationality, 1974–1994. *Population Studies, 59*, 71–85.

Kang Fu, V. (2008). Interracial-Interethnic Unions and Fertility in the United States. *Journal of Marriage and Family, 70*(3), 783–95.

Kibria, N. (2002). *Becoming Asian American.* Baltimore: Johns Hopkins University Press.

Lee, S. M., & Edmonston, B. (2005). New marriages, new families: US racial and Hispanic intermarriage. *Population Bulletin, 60*(1), 1–38.

Leslie, L. A., & Letiecq, B. L. (2004). Marital quality of African American and White partners in interracial couples. *Personal Relationships, 11*(4), 559–74.

Lichter, D. T., Qian, Z., & Mellott, L. M. (2006). Marriage or dissolution? Union transitions among poor cohabiting women. *Demography, 43*(2), 223–40.

Livingston, G., & Brown, A. (2017). Intermarriage in the U.S. 50 Years After *Loving v. Virginia. Pew Research Center.* Retrieved October 1, 2021. https://www.pewresearch.org/social-trends/2017/05/18/intermarriage-in-the-u-s-50-years-after-loving-v-virginia/.

Lundquist, J. H. (2006). The Black-White gap in marital dissolution among young adults: What can a counterfactual scenario tell us? *Social Problems, 53*(3), 421–41.

Miller, B. (2020). Black interracial families in U.S. society. In A. James (ed), *Black Families: A Systems approach* (pp. 88–96). San Diego, CA: Cognella Press.

Millward, J. (2010). "The relics of slavery": Interracial sex and manumission in the American south. *Frontiers, 31*(3), 22–30,145. Retrieved from http://csulb.idm.oclc.org/login?url=https://search-proquest-com.csulb.idm.oclc.org/docview/822042548?accountid=10351.

Newport, F. (2013). In U.S., 87% Approve of Black-White Marriage, v. 4% in 1958. *Gallup.* Retrieved from http://www.gallup.com/poll/163697/approve-marriage-blacks-whites.aspx.

Ono, H., & Berg, J. (2010). Homogamy and intermarriage of Japanese and Japanese Americans with Whites surrounding World War II. *Journals of Marriage and Family, 72*, 1249–62.

Passl, J., Wang, W., & Taylor, P. (2010). Marrying Out: One-in-Seven New U.S. Marriages Is Interracial or Interethnic." *Pew Research Center's Social & Demographic Trends Project.*

Pew Research Center. (2017). *Intermarriage in the U.S. 50 Years After Loving v. Virginia.* Retrieved from https://www.pewsocialtrends.org/2017/05/18/intermarriage-in-the-u-s-50-years-after-loving-v-virginia/.

Qian, Z., & Lichter, D. T. (2011). Changing Patterns of Interracial Marriage in a MultiracialSociety. *Journal of Marriage and Family, 73*(5), 1065–84.

Roy, R. N. (2019). Transition to Parenthood. In R. N. Roy & A. Rollins, (2019). *Biracial Families: Crossing Boundaries, Blending Cultures, and Challenging Racial Ideologies.* (pp. 105–27). New York, NY: Springer.

Roy, R. N. & Rollins, A. (2019). *Biracial Families: Crossing Boundaries, Blending Cultures, and Challenging Racial Ideologies.* New York, NY: Springer.

Troy, A. B., Lewis-Smith, J., & Laurenceau, J. P. (2006). Interracial and intraracial romantic relationships: The search for differences in satisfaction, conflict, and attachment style. *Journal of Social and Personal Relationships, 23*(1), 65–80.

Wang, W. (2012). The rise of intermarriage: Rates, characteristics vary by race and gender. *Social and Demographic Trends.* Washington, D.C.: Pew Research Center.

Wang, H., Kao, G., & Joyner, K. (2006). Stability of interracial and intraracial romantic relationships among adolescents. *Social Science Research, 35*(2), 435–53.

Webb, F. J., Burrell, J., & Jefferson, S. G. (2019). Social constitutionality of race in America: Some meanings for bi/multiracial families. In R. Nazarinia Roy & A. Rollins (Eds.), *Biracial families: Crossing boundaries, blending cultures, and challenging racial ideologies* (pp. 9–32). New York, NY: Springer.

Wolfe, B. (2015). Racial Integrity Laws (1924–1930). *Encyclopedia Virginia.* Retrieved July 1, 2020 (https://www.encyclopediavirginia.org/Racial_Integrity _Laws_of_the_1920s).

Yancey G. (2007). Experiencing Racism: Differences in the Experiences of Whites Married to Blacks and Non-Black Racial Minorities. *Journal of Comparative Family Studies, 38*(2), 197–213.

Zhang, Y., & Van Hook, J. (2009). Marital dissolution among interracial couples. *Journal of Marriage and Family, 71*(1), 95–107.

Chapter 1

Bridging the Interracial Literature

CHAPTER OVERVIEW

A bridge is a means of connection or transition (Merriam-Webster.com, 2020), often pertaining to something joining land masses (e.g., Golden Gate Bridge) or points in space-time (e.g., Einstein-Rosen Bridge). As a sociologist, I conceptualize people as *social bridges* who connect individuals, groups, institutions, organizations, social networks, and other elements of society across space-time. In diverse societies like the United States, social bridges are key actors that link people with different socio-demographic backgrounds (e.g., race, social class, gender) that may otherwise remain disconnected.

In terms of race and romantic relationships, most people have their first romantic experience by age eighteen (Brown, 2004; Collins & van Dulme, 2006; Joyner & Udry, 2000), and although the majority of people choose to be in same-race relationships (SRRs) with partners who share the same racial identity as him- or herself, more and more young adults are forming interracial relationships (IRRs) (Jones, 2005; Joyner & Kao, 2005; Newport, 2013; Pew Research Center, 2015; Yancey, 2002). Those individuals who do cross racial lines for romance function as social bridges that directly or indirectly connect their families, friends, communities, racial groups, and the broader society through their interracial partnerships. Generation after generation, young adults (ages 13–29) are most likely to engage in IRRs and serve as the social bridges connecting their racially diverse networks. Those young adults from each generation that willingly connect people from different racial groups through their own interracial romantic involvement are referred to as the *Bridge Kids*.

Given that the acceptance and prevalence of IRRs can be seen as a valuable indicator of a society's race relations (Gordon, 1964), the prevalence of such relationships among the Bridge Kids might serve as a predictor for the future of race relations. Moreover, to fully comprehend the impact IRRs are having on our society, as well as the impact society has on IRRs, requires an examination of the personal and social factors that affect the lives and well-being of those in mixed-race partnerships. With this in mind, the purpose of this book is to use the existing literature to bring greater attention to the personal and social factors that affect the lives and well-being of the people in interracial relationships, especially young adults. The intention of this specific chapter is to provide a general discussion for how trends in the prevalence and approval of IRRs impact the lives and well-being of the Bridge Kids and others in IRRs, as well as highlight the advantages of approaching this complex social issue using an interdisciplinary approach grounded in a sociological framework.

INTERRACIAL ROMANTIC RELATIONSHIPS

Ever since the anti-miscegenation laws that prohibited interracial romantic relationships were deemed unconstitutional by the Supreme Court in 1967 (*Loving vs. Virginia* 388 U.S. 1, 1967), there has been a precipitous rise in the number of interracially married (intermarried) people in the United States (U.S.). Now, more people than ever are crossing racial lines and becoming romantically involved in interracial relationships (IRRs) evidenced by the prevalence of intermarriage growing from roughly 300,000 (less than 1 percent of all marriages) in 1970 to over 11 million (10 percent of all marriages) in 2015 (Lee & Edmonston, 2005; Livingston & Brown, 2017). There are no signs that intermarriage rates will be slowing down any time soon because 17 percent of people who were newly married within the past year did so interracially (Livingston & Brown, 2017). To put this trend into better perspective, the current intermarriage rate is a staggering 1,700 percent increase since their legalization in 1967. When considering less formally recognized partnerships, 17 percent of cohabiting adults are in interracial relationships (Pew Research Center 2017), and approximately 17 percent of romantically involved adolescents are interracially dating (Kreager, 2008; Miller 2014; Vaquero & Kao, 2005). In other words, over the past fifty years, the United States has seen the prevalence of interracial relationships surge from about 1 out of every 100 partnerships to nearly 1 in 5.

The increasing prevalence of interracial romance has assuredly been influenced by the mainstream media and pop culture's more frequent depictions of mixed-race couples and their families. Beginning in 1951, when the *I Love Lucy* show made Lucille Ball and Desi Arnaz the first interracial couple featured on a television series, the media has grown more comfortable showing interracial couples and their romantic encounters. Over the years, the number and frequency of IRRs portrayed by the media has significantly grown, including, but in no way limited to, Captain Kirk's kiss of Lieutenant Nyota Uhura in *Star Trek* (1968), Tom and Helen Willis in *The Jeffersons* (1975), as well as Jay and Gloria Pritchett in *Modern Family* (2009). The experiences of interracial couples have also been prominently featured in big-screen movies like *Look Who's Coming to Dinner* (1967), *Jungle Fever* (1991), *Save the Last Dance* (2001), and *Loving* (2016). The holistic experiences of interracial couples along with their Multiracial families have been portrayed more recently in television shows such as *Keeping Up with the Kardashians* (2007) and *Mixed-ish* (2019), as well as the movie *Cheaper by the Dozen* (2022). Additionally, there are numerous celebrities in IRRs who have Multiracial families, like Eva Mendes (Hispanic) and her husband, Ryan Gosling (White); Serena Williams (Black) and her husband, Alexis Ohanian (White); as well as Rachel Meghan Markle, Duchess of Sussex (Black-White) and her husband, Prince Henry "Harry" Charles Albert David Duke of Sussex (White). In this fashion, popular culture has undoubtedly helped people learn to view IRRs and their Multiracial families as a socially normative part our society.

The idea that pop culture and other factors has helped destigmatize interracial involvement is supported by the analysis of trend data depicting a positive correlation between the increasing rates of IRRs and the social acceptance of such relationships (McCarthy, 2021). On multiple occasions over the past century, nationally representative Gallup polls have asked their participants the question "Do you approve or disapprove of marriage between Black people and White people?" Only 4 percent of Americans approved in 1920; 20 percent in 1967 (the year interracial relationships became legal), and approval reached an all-time high with 94 percent approving in 2021 (McCarthy, 2021). That means there has been a complete shift in attitudes as one hundred years ago, 96 percent of Americans disapproved of intermarriage, and now nearly that same amount approves of them. Moreover, not only does an overwhelming percentage of Americans say they approve of intermarriage, the percentage that believes interracial marriage "generally is a good thing for our society" rose from 24 percent in 2010 to 39 percent in 2019, whereas the proportion that view intermarriage as "a bad thing" fell from 13 percent to 9 percent during this same time frame (Pew Research Center, 2019). Taken together, these data show increasingly more people approve of IRRs and believe they are good for society while fewer people see them as bad, which is indicative of a positive trend that implies Americans have become more open-minded towards interracial romance.

When asked about their attitudes for approving the intermarriage of a family member however, the results of a Pew Research Center survey were less positive. Partner acceptability significantly varies by race, as intermarriage to a White partner is seen as most acceptable by 81 percent of the U.S. population, followed by an Asian partner (75 percent), Hispanic partner (73 percent), and having a Black partner (66 percent) is seen as least acceptable (Passel, Wang, & Taylor 2010). This means Americans are generally okay with the idea of intermarriage until it involves their own family members, and even then, acceptance depends on the race of the potential partner. This sentiment is reflected in the work of Herman and Campbell (2012) titled "*I wouldn't but you can: Attitudes towards interracial relationships,*" which found White women are "more likely to reject interracial relationships with Blacks for themselves, although not for others" (353). The racial variation in interracial partner acceptability is important because the *assimilation theory* presupposes partners and couples that are less socially accepted, tend to experience more oppositional treatment and stigmatization (Gordon, 1964). Consequently, it is likely that, based on the couple's racial composition (e.g., White-Asian, Asian-Hispanic, Hispanic-Black), people in different interracial partnerships do not share the same lived experiences. Since these data show that Americans are generally more accepting of racial minorities with White partners than Whites with minority partners, implies interracially involved minorities that have a White partner may be viewed more favorably and have better social experiences than Whites coupled with any minority but especially Blacks.

Upon further reflection of the data, one must step back from the canvas to clearly see the picture that has been painted. Despite the 94 percent approval rating of Black-White intermarriage generally, public views of Black persons as the least acceptable interracial partner for one's own family member is much too significant to overlook because Black-White relationships have long been the "standard candle" for measuring interracial romance and race relations in the United States. It is particularly interesting to note that, although the prevalence of IRRs is thought to reflect a society's race relations and beliefs regarding the acceptance of minority groups into the mainstream society (Bogardus, 1947; Gordon, 1964), approval rates of Black-White interracial couples do not mirror contemporary attitudes for race relations.

For instance, data from a nationally representative Gallup poll on *U.S. Approval of Marriage Between Black People and White People* shows that, between the years 2013 and 2021, approval of Black-White intermarriage in the United States rose from 87 percent to an all-time high of 94 percent (McCarthy, 2021), which would seemingly suggest race relations between the two groups is very good. A different Gallup poll measuring attitudes toward race relations between White and Black people, however, reveals that during the same period (2013–2021), the proportion of Americans that viewed White-Black race relations as either "somewhat good" or "very good" dropped from 70 percent in 2013 to a modern-day low of about 37 percent in 2021 (Gallup, 2022). In light of this paradox, whereby society is express-ing its overwhelming approval of interracial romance in the backdrop of a social climate with contentious race relations, it seems imperative to explore the broader impact IRRs are having on race relations as well as explore the effects race relations are having on the lives and well-being of people in IRRs.

A deeper dive into explaining this paradox is necessary because, on one hand, the trends in rising approval of IRRs contrasted by the declining race relations could be due to people's beliefs that interracial relationships are good, in spite of the poor state of race relations in America. For instance, given the numerous race riots and racial protests that occurred from 2014 to 2020 (Rowen & Chamberlain), it is highly probable for someone to view contemporary race relations as poor and at the same time approve of IRRs and even believe they are good for society, especially if that person supports having racial equality in our society. Similarly, for numerous personal and broader societal reasons, even people in IRRs themselves may approve of interracial romance but still perceive today's race relations as being very bad.

Another premise for explaining this contradiction could be that people say, and possibly believe, they support mixed-race relationships when in fact either consciously or unconsciously, they do not. The rationale for this proposal stems from research by Skinner and Hudac (2017) who found, using a sample of Whites (87 percent) and Nonwhites (13 percent), that most Nonblack people outwardly express acceptance of interracial romance by communicating their own willingness to interracially date, live with, marry, and even have a child with someone who is Black. Yet, when those same Nonblack people were shown images of Black-Black, White-White, and Black-White couples, the photos of Black-White interracial couples were much more likely to stimulate an *insula activation response* in their brain. An insula activation reflects perceiving stimuli as a potential risk or threat (Preuschoff, Quartz, & Bossaerts, 2008) that elicits an emotional reaction associated with feelings of disgust and, in this case, dehumanizing percep-tions of people in IRRs. The Skinner and Hudac (2017) study therefore shows that some people might say they approve of IRRs, when deep down they do not. Accordingly, even among people that outwardly convey acceptance for interracial romance, it is possible they still have derogatory perceptions of interracial couples that contribute to their antisocial behavior toward people in IRRs that can adversely affect the lives and well-being of those in mixed-race relationships.

ROMANTIC RELATIONSHIPS AND
RACIAL DISPARITIES IN HEALTH

Regardless of whether someone is in a same-race or an interracial relationship, most romantically involved people want to live a long and healthy life with their partner. Romantic partnerships have shown to encourage positive health behaviors for both partners including eating healthier, reduced drug and alcohol use, and better health maintenance with more frequent visits to the physician to maintain their health (Duncan, Wilkerson, & England, 2006), which contribute to married men and women having a higher life expectancy (i.e., live longer) than their unmarried peers (Borella, DeNardi, & Yang, 2016; Harvard Health, 2019). These health advantages are at least partially related to romantic partnerships being social relationships that provide people with important resources to cope with enduring daily stressors (Benin & Keith, 1995) as well as physical and mental health issues (Cohen, Underwood & Gottlieb, 2000; Lincoln, 2000). Romantic relationships also provide some people with economic resources and personal resources like happiness that may cultivate better mental health, which is also linked to reports of better physical health (Waite and Gallagher 2000; Waite and Lehrer 2003; Umberson & Montez, 2010). In these ways, romantic partnerships commonly provide a multitude of health-related benefits to men and women from all racial backgrounds.

For some people, however, romantic relationships are sources of stress and poor health. For instance, relationships with intimate partner violence can create toxic environments that have numerous harmful effects on one's mental, physical, and social well-being (Lau et al., 2019; Miller & Irvin, 2017; Ogbe et al., 2020). Relationships between, or including, members of marginalized groups such as sexual minorities in the lesbian, gay, bisexual, transgender (LBGT) community, those with physical disabilities, or racial minorities can also be sources of stress for one or both partners. Moreover, since the individuals in a romantic relationship are not in a socially isolated vacuum, it is likely that some of the experiences and resources that affect the well-being of one person also affects the life and well-being of their partner, especially if one partner is a member of a marginalized group. It is therefore unlikely that the health benefits of romantic relationships are fundamentally equal for everyone, which makes it important to consider the bi-directional influence of both partners on one another's well-being to gain a more holistic view of the association between romantic relationship status and health.

One factor that appears to have a significant bi-directional influence on the lives and well-being of romantically involved persons is the racial background of each partner. The importance of this distinction should not be underestimated because, despite the growing number of people who are engaging in interracial romance, researchers have predominately focused on the health of individuals in same-race romantic relationships (SRRs). However, a small but growing body of literature shows that, compared to those in SRRs, people in IRRs generally have poorer psychological well-being (Bratter & Eschbach, 2006; Kroeger & Williams, 2011; Miller, 2014; Tillman & Miller, 2017), poorer social well-being (Bell & Hastings, 2015; Tillman & Miller, 2017), and lower overall self-rated health (Barr & Simons, 2014; Yu & Zhang, 2017). Collectively, the findings of the extant literature support the suggestion by Miller (2014) that interracial relationships may be viewed as a social stressor in and of themselves and as such, by virtue of having a partner with a different racial background, many people in IRRs have an increased vulnerability to disease and illnesses.

The implicit and explicit opposition faced by people in IRRs from the millions of Americans that disapprove of interracial relationships and do not believe they are good for society (Pew Research Center, 2017), is a social stressor that likely contributes to the poorer health and well-being reported by people in IRRs. For example, at the individual level, people in interracial partnerships report experiencing racism, discrimination, and stigmatization from family, friends, and the general society for being in a mixed-race relationship (Bell & Hastings, 2011; Edmonds & Killen, 2009; Seshadri & Knudson-Martin, 2013; Silvestrini, 2020; Solsberry, 1994; Steinbugler, 2014). Specific instances of such mistreatment include parents disowning their children for dating someone outside their racial group (Bell & Hastings, 2015), a justice of the peace refusing to lawfully wed mixed-race partners (CNN.com, 2009), and an interracial couple being physically attacked that resulted in the stabbing of one partner (Wootson, 2016). All the perpetrators in these and many other instances specifically referenced their opposition to interracial romance as the driving force behind their spiteful actions.

Exposure to social stressors like racism, discrimination, and stigmatization have been shown to adversely affect people's life satisfaction, health, and well-being (Broudy et al., 2007; T. Brown et al., 2000; Gee et al., 2007; Kessler, Mickelson, & Williams, 1999; Miller, Rote, & Keith, 2013; Prelow, Mosher, & Bowman, 2006). As such, instead of being less taboo, as many people suggest, crossing racial borders for romance may actually lead to what I refer to as a *partner penalty* for some people whose well-being is adversely affected by their interracial relationship (Bratter & Eschbach, 2006, Miller, 2014; Miller & Tillman, 2017). Alternatively, given the general benefits of romantic partnerships for well-being (Simon, 2002; Williams & Umberson, 2004), some interracially involved people receive a *partner premium* whereby they report having better health than their counterparts in same-race relationships (Miller et al., 2022; Miller & Kail, 2016). However, researchers are still trying to gain a clearer picture of how involvement in interracial relationships affects a person's health and well-being.

The inclusion of the Bridge Kids is necessary to acquire a more comprehensive understanding of the association between interracial romance and health for several notable reasons. For one, young adults face an elevated risk of having poorer mental health than their older counterparts. In fact, among the 52.9 million adults with a mental illness, those ages eighteen to twenty-five have the highest prevalence (30.6 percent) of being diagnosed with a mental illness in the past year, which is contrasted by them having the lowest rates of receiving mental health services (42.1 percent) (NIMH.gov, 2022). This means that less than half of the sixteen million young adults with a diagnosed mental illness are being treated. As a result, young adults like the Bridge Kids are most likely to engage in interracial romance *and* suffer from the types of mental illness that can seriously impair their lives and well-being. The length of these impairments may be substantial however, considering a person's well-being during young adulthood is a significant predictor for their well-being later in life (Frech, 2012; Lewinsohn et al., 2003), and the literature currently indicates interracial romance is generally associated with poorer health outcomes for both adolescents and adults (Barr & Simons, 2014; Bratter & Eschbach, 2006; Miller, 2014; Tillman & Miller, 2017; Wong & Penner, 2018). For these reasons, incorporating the Bridge Kids into the romantic relationship and health discourse will provide a new perspective to help us better discern the social determinants that negatively and positively impact the well-being of people in both same-race and interracial romantic relationships across the life course.

In addition, and perhaps more importantly, examining the partner selection process and well-being of the Bridge Kids can provide families, researchers, teachers, clinicians, and health practitioners with a new and extraordinary lens for examining current health trends and predicting future health outcomes. Moreover, becoming familiar with the well-being of the Bridge Kids can greatly improve our overall comprehension of the observed racial disparities in health, as well as the association between couple's racial composition and health across the life course. Doing so can also provide us with much greater insight on the effect race relations have on the lives and well-being of people in IRRs as well as the influence IRRs are having on race relations. To effectively use such a powerful lens as a tool for social evaluation, requires an innovative approach for conceptualizing race, race relations, and interracial romance.

THE SOCIOLOGICAL IMAGINATION

Taking a holistic approach to address such a complex social issue like the association between interracial romance and well-being, necessitates an individual having an open-minded approach like using his or her sociological imagination. The *sociological imagination* is a term coined by the sociologist C. Wright Mills (1959) in reference to a person's ability to examine social issues from an unbiased perspective that recognizes people's lives are conditioned by socially structured institutions like family, education, the government, and health care. People can then impartially view others and broader issues by imagining how their own life compares to those with different social characteristics (e.g., race, gender, social class) or in different social circumstances (e.g., neighborhood, job, social environment) than their self. Put another way, the sociological imagination helps people recognize the differential impact social institutions have on the attitudes, behaviors, and choices of people in our society.

Developing one's sociological imagination also entails taking a person's socio-historical perspective into account. This means acknowledging that as social institutions change over time, people's attitudes, behaviors, and opportunities change, as well. This is especially salient concerning issues related to racial identity, race relations, and interracial romance. For example, when using the sociological imagination, a person can envisage why race relations change over time, how attitudes towards interracial romance vary by generations, how racial identity influences the way people label relationships as either SRRs or IRRs, or why people approve of interracial romance with some racial groups and not others. Therefore, based on the social contexts of the given timeframe, the sociological imagination is a theoretical tool that allows people to better understand the beliefs and behaviors of individuals and groups by figuratively "putting themselves in someone else's shoes" (Mills, 1959).

Mills (1959) also posited the sociological imagination involves recognizing that many issues people see as their own private problems are actually public issues because they are shared by many people. That is, if "certain problems are shared by groups of people, they may have a common cause and be best dealt with through collective action" (Germov, 2019: p. 5). This specifically applies to those in IRRs because many people in mixed-race partnerships: (1) are stigmatized and discriminated against; and (2) appear to be more vulnerable to health problems than those in same-race relationships. That means the personal troubles shared by the millions of individuals in mixed-race partnerships that adversely impact their lives and well-being, probably have common causes that require the collective action of the general public, and not just those in IRRs, to best address the underlying issues affecting their well-being and social experiences. As such, examining the health of people in interracial relationships is a critically important public health matter and using the sociological imagination—recognizing these issues are shared by millions of people and truly putting oneself in their metaphorical shoes to understand how they are affected—is paramount to improving our understanding of this social issue.

THE INTERSECTIONALITY OF COUPLE'S RACIAL COMPOSITION

In addition to the use of one's sociological imagination, comprehending the complexities associated with IRRs warrants a novel theoretical approach. For example, the existing research clearly demonstrates the health and well-being for individuals in IRRs is impacted by the synergistic effects of the person's race *and* gender as well as the race of his or her partner (Bratter & Eschbach, 2006; Miller & Kail, 2016; Miller et al., 2022; Wong & Penner, 2018). These studies generally show that interracial romance does not affect everyone's health in the same ways, but rather some people benefit from interracial partnerships whereas others do not, and these health disparities largely differ by race and gender. However, because individuals in IRRs have predominantly been excluded from the health disparities literature until relatively recently, determining the underlying factors associated with these differences requires the traditional approaches for this topic be re-envisioned using an analytical framework that specifically addresses the unparalleled experiences of interracial couples. It is for this reason that *intertersectionality*, which refers to examining variations in the multiplicative effects of two or more social statuses on an outcome (Crenshaw, 1989), is a useful theoretical framework to analyze the interconnection between race, gender, and partner's race for persons in IRRs.

Kimberle Crenshaw more recently stated that intersectionality "is a lens through which you can see where power comes and collides, where it interlocks and intersects. It's not simply that there's a race problem here, a gender problem here, and a class or LBGTQ problem there. Many times that framework erases what happens to people who are subject to all of these things (Columbia.edu, 2017)." Because these same "problems" extend to the characteristics of romantically involved persons, I propose it can be argued that inequalities in power and status contribute to differential experiences among men and women based on their *relationship type* (same-race or interracial).

For example, Crenshaw (1989) argued that since White people and men have more power and privileges than both Nonwhite people and women respectively, Black women (being Nonwhite *and* female) are particularly disadvantaged in terms of power and privilege, and therefore have different experiences than both White women and Black men. This example illustrates that people with the same social position (e.g., race or gender) do not necessarily have the same social experiences, and we gain a much better understanding of these differences when accounting for the multiplicative effects of more than just one social position. When extrapolating this argument to consider both partners in a heterosexual Black-White IRR for example, it is likely the experiences of this interracial pairing vary by the intersection of race and gender (race*gender) such that we see observable differences for: 1) a Black woman partnered with a White man compared to a Black man partnered with a White woman; 2) a Black woman partnered with a White man compared to a White woman partnered with a Black man; 3) a Black man partnered with a White woman compared to a White man partnered with a Black woman; and 4) a White woman partnered with a Black man compared to a White man partnered with a Black woman. It is along these lines that the intersectionality lens can be used to assess how the experiences of romantically involved individuals vary by the couple's racial composition consisting of a person's race and gender as well as their partner's race. The interaction

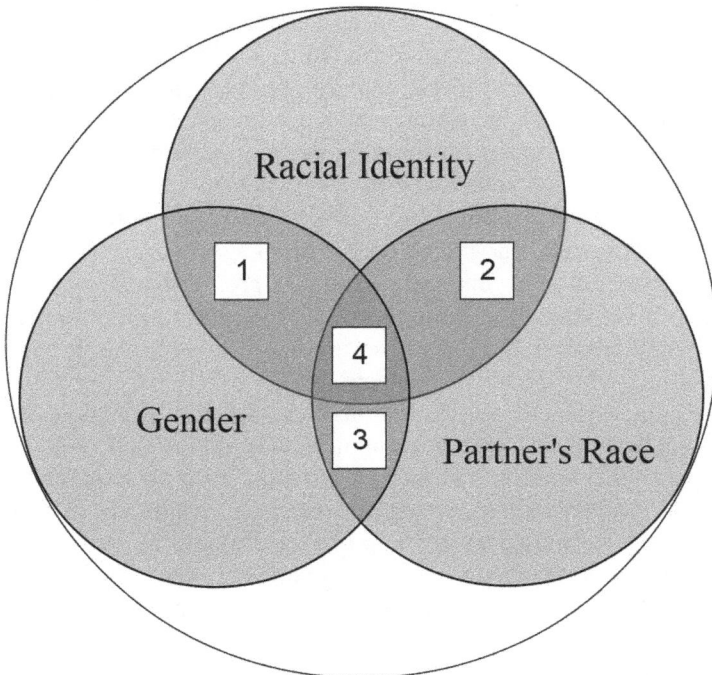

Figure 1.1. Intersectionality of Couple's Racial Composition. Created by the author.

of these couple characteristics is visually depicted in Figure 1.1, showing the combined effects of: (1) a person's race and gender; (2) a person's race and their partner's race; (3) a person's gender and their partner's race; and (4) a person's race and gender as well as their partner's race.

THE BRIDGE KIDS AND SOCIAL CHANGE

Using the sociological imagination, some social scientists, including myself, view the prevalence of IRRs as a measure of a society's racial ideology and its acceptance of racial assimilation (Gordon, 1964; Joyner & Kao, 2005; Kennedy, 2003; Miller, 2014). This perspective presumes that a racially diverse society with anti-miscegenation policies that allows little to no interracial romance, inherently has issues with racism, whereas a diverse society without such laws *and* a high prevalence of IRRs will have fewer issues related to racism. In the United States, the contemporary increase of racial integration into the residential, educational, and employment sectors are indicative of cultural assimilation, but interracial relationships and inter-marriages imply an even higher level of structural assimilation and a more egalitarian racial ideology (Gordon, 1964; Miller & Kail, 2016). Thus, the increasing commonality of IRRs appear to reflect a degree of social change in U.S. race relations and the American family.

Although reluctance to social change and interracial romance remain prominent issues, the desire to improve U.S. race relations continues and is evidenced by the nationwide protests throughout 2020 that called for greater social justice and racial equality (Rowen & Chamberlain, 2022). The Racial Protests of 2020 were spurred by several high-profile police shootings of unarmed Black people, and united people of all ages, genders, racial groups, and skin tones for one common cause: the promotion of racial equality through social change. The protestors clearly recognized the role race con-tinues to play in our society and used their collective voice to address the ever-lingering public problem of racism.

Many young adults today are bastions of social change. This undoubtedly includes the Bridge Kids who are changing society in their own way by bridg-ing race relations, bridging families and friends, bridging communities, and bridging our understanding of racial disparities in health. The Bridge Kids are also redefining our understanding of race and are the catalyst for more people forming racially diverse social networks that have meaningful social interactions. Many of these connections are of a romantic nature, which lead to the formation of interracial families and contribute to the biracial baby boom, which in and of itself is having a profound effect on race relations as well as altering people's perceptions of racial identity. As such, the pervasive impact of the Bridge Kids warrants a closer investigation into their influence on society as well as society's impact on them.

REFERENCES

Barr, A. B., & Simons, R. L. (2014). A Dyadic Analysis of Relationships and Health: Does Couple-level Context Condition Partner Effects?" *Journal of Family Psychology, 28*(4), 448–59.

Bell, G. C., & Hastings, S. O. (2011). Black and White interracial couples: Managing relational disapproval through facework. Howard Journal of Communications, 22(3), 240–59.

Bell, G. C., & Hastings, S. O. (2015). Exploring Parental Approval and Disapproval for Black and White Interracial Couples. *Journal of Social Issues, 71*(4), 755–71.

Benin, M., & Keith, V. (1995). The social support of employed African and anglo mothers.*Journal of Family Issues, 16*(3), 275–97.

Bogardus, E. S. 1947. Measurement of personal-group relations. *Sociometry, 10*, 306–11.

Borella, M., DeNardi, M., & Yang, F. (2016). Gender, Marriage, and Life Expectancy. *National Bureau of Economic Research*, Working Paper No. 22817.

Bratter, J., & Eschbach, K. (2006). What about the couple? Interracial marriage and psychological distress. Social Science Research, 35, 1025–47.

Broudy, R., Brondolo, E., Coakley, V., Brady, N., Cassells, A., Tobin, J. N., & Sweeney, M. (2006). Perceived Ethnic Discrimination in Relation to Daily Moods and Negative Social Interactions. *Journal of Behavioral Medicine* 30(1), 31–43.

Brown, B. Bradford. 2004. "Adolescents' relationships with peers." Handbook of Adolescent Psychology, 2nd edition. Richard M. Lerner and Laurence Steinberg, editors. Wiley, 363–94.

Cohen, S., Gottlieb, B. H., & Underwood. L. G. (2000). Social relationships and health. In S. Cohen, L. G. Underwood, & B. H. Gottlieb (Eds.), Social support measurement and intervention: A guide for health and social scientists. Oxford University Press, 3–25.

Collins, W. Andrew., and Van Dulmen, Manfred. 2006. "'The course of true love(s) . . . ': Origins and pathways in the development of romantic relationships." *Romance and sex in adolescence and emerging adulthood: Risks and opportunities*. Ann Crouter and Alan Booth, editors. Lawrence Erlbaum Associates, 63–86.

Columbia Law School. (2017, June 8). *Kimberle' Crenshaw on Intersectionality, More Than Two Decades Later.* https://www.law.columbia.edu/news/archive/ kimberle-crenshaw- intersectionality-more-two-decades-later.

CNN.com. (2009, November 3). *Louisiana justice who refused interracial marriage resigns. CNN.* http://www.cnn.com/2009/US/11/03/louisiana.interracial.marriage/ index.html.

Crenshaw, K. (1989). Demarginalizing the Intersection of Race and Sex: A Black Feminist Critique of Antidiscrimination Doctrine, Feminist 4eory and Antiracist

Politics. *University of Chicago Legal Forum, 1* (Article 8). h5p://chicagounbound. uchicago.edu/uclf/vol1989/iss1/8.

Duncan, G. J., Wilkerson, B., England. P. (2006). Cleaning up their act: the effects of marriage and cohabitation on licit and illicit drug use. *Demography 43*(4), 691–710.

Edmonds, C., & Killen, M. (2009). Do Adolescent's Perceptions of Parental Racial Attitudes Relate to Their Intergroup Contact and Cross-Race Relationships?. *Group Processes & Intergroup Relations, 12(1)*, 5–21.

Frech A. (2012). Healthy Behavior Trajectories between Adolescence and Young Adulthood. *Advances in life course research, 17*(2), 59–68.

Gallup. (2022). Race Relations. *Gallup.* https://news.gallup.com/poll/1687/race -relations.aspx.

Gee, G., Spencer, M., Chen, J., Yip, T., & Takeuchi, D. (2007). The Association between Self-Reported Racial Discrimination and 12-month DSM-IV Mental Disorders among AsianAmericans Nationwide. *Social Science and Medicine, 64*(10), 1984–96.

Germov, J. (2019). Imagining health problems as social issues. In J. Germov (Ed.), *An introduction to health sociology*. Oxford University Press, 2–23.

Gordon, M. (1964). *Assimilation in American Life: The Role of Race, Religion, and National Origin.* Oxford University Press.

Harvard Health Publishing. (2019, June 5). *Marriage and men's health.* https://www .health.harvard.edu/mens-health/marriage-and-mens-health.

Herman, M. R., & Campbell, M. E. (2012). I wouldn't but you can: Attitudes towards interracial relationships. *Social Science Research, 41*, 343–58.

Jones, J. M. (2005, October 7). Most Americans Approve of Interracial Dating. *Gallup.* http://www.gallup.com/poll/19033/Most-Americans-Approve-Interracial -Dating.aspx.

Joyner, K., & Kao, G. (2005). Interracial Relationships and the Transition to Adulthood. *American Sociological Review, 70*, 563–81.

Joyner, Kara, and Richard J. Udry. (2000). "You Don't Bring Me Anything but Down: Adolescent Romance and Depression." *Journal of Health and Social and Behavior* 41:369–91.

Kennedy, R. (2003). *Interracial intimacies: Sex, marriage, identity, and adoption.* New York, NY: Pantheon Books.

Kessler, R. C., Mickelson, K., & Williams, D. (1999). The Prevalence, Distribution, and Mental Health Correlates of Perceived Discrimination in the United States. *Journal of Health and Social Behavior, 40*(3), 208–30.

Kreager, D. (2008). Guarded Borders: Adolescent Interracial Romance and Peer Trouble at School. *Social Forces, 87*(2), 887–910.

Kroeger, R., & Williams, K. (2011). Consequences of Black Exceptionalism? Interracial Unions with Blacks, Depressive Symptoms, and Relationship Satisfaction. *The Sociological Quarterly*, 52, 400–20.

Lau, K. K. H., Randall, A. K., Duran, N. D., & Tao, C. (2019). Examining the Effects of Couples' Real-Time Stress and Coping Processes on Interaction Quality: Language Use as a Mediator. *Frontiers in Psychology, 9* (January), 1–14.

Lee, S., & Edmonston, B. (2005). New Marriages, New Families: U.S. Racial and Hispanic Intermarriage. *Population Bulletin, 60*(2), 3–36.

Lewinsohn, P. M., Klein, D. N., Durbin, E. C., Seeley, J.R., & Rohde, P. (2003). Family study of subthreshold depressive symptoms: risk factor for MDD? *Journal of Affective Disorders, 77*(2), 149–57.

Lincoln, K. D. (2000). Social Support, Negative Social Interactions, and Psychological Well-being. *Social Service Review, 74*(2), 231–52.

Livingston, G., & Brown, A. (2017). Intermarriage in the U.S. 50 Years after *Loving v. Virginia. Pew Research Center.* Retrieved October 1, 2021. (https:// www.pewresearch.org/social- trends/2017/05/18/intermarriage-in-the-u-s-50-years -after-loving-v-virginia/).

Loving v. Virginia, 388 U.S. 1 (1967).

McCarthy, J. (2021, September 10). U.S. Approval of Interracial Marriage at New High of 94%. *Gallup.* https://news.gallup.com/poll/354638/approval-interracial -marriage-new-high.aspx?version=print.

Merriam-Webster Dictionary. (2020). *Bridge.* https://www.merriamwebster.com/ dictionary/bridge.

Miller, B. (2014). What are the odds: An examination of adolescent interracial romance and risk for depression. *Youth & Society, 49*(2), 180–202.

Miller, B., & Irvin, J. (2017). Invisible Scars: Comparing the Mental Health of LGB and Heterosexual Intimate Partner Violence Survivors. *Journal of Homosexuality, 64*(9), 1180–95.

Miller, B., James, A., & Roy, R. N. (2022). Loving Across Racial Lines: Associations between Gender and Partner Race and the Health of Young Adults. *Journal of Child and Family Studies, 31*(2), 703–15.

Miller, B., & Kail, B. L. (2016). Exploring the effects of spousal race on the self-rated health of intermarried adults. Sociological Perspectives, 59(3), 604–618.

Miller, B., Rote, S., & Keith, V. (2013). Coping with Racial Discrimination: Assessing the Vulnerability of African Americans and the Mediated Moderation of Psychosocial Resources. *Society and Mental Health, 3*(2), 133–50.

Mills, C. W. (1959). *The sociological imagination.* New York: Oxford University Press

National Institute of Mental Health. (2022, January). *Mental Illness.* https://www .nimh.nih.gov/health/statistics/mental-illness.

Newport, F. (2013, July 25). In U.S., 87% Approve of Black-White Marriage, v. 4% in 1958. *Gallup.* http://www.gallup.com/poll/163697/approve-marriage-blacks -whites.aspx.

Ogbe, E., Harmon, S., Van den Bergh, R., & Degomme, O. (2020). A systematic review of intimate partner violence interventions focused on improving social sup- port and/mental health outcomes of survivors. *PLOS ONE, June: 1–27.*

Passel, J., Wang, W., & Taylor, P. (2010, June 4). Marrying Out: One-in-Seven New U.S. Marriages Is Interracial or Interethnic. *Pew Research Center's Social & Demographic Trends Project.* https://www.pewresearch.org/social-trends/2010/06 /04/marrying-out/.

mente

Pew Research Center. (2015). *What Census Calls Us: A Historical Timeline.* https://www.pewsocialtrends.org/wp-content/uploads/sites/3/2015/06/ST_15.06.11_MultiRacial-Timeline.pdf.

Pew Research Center. (2017). *Intermarriage in the U.S. 50 Years After* Loving v. Virginia. http://www.pewsocialtrends.org/2017/05/18/intermarriage-in-the-u-s-50-years-after-loving-v-virginia/.

Pew Research Center. (2019, April). *Race in America.* https://www.pewresearch.org/social-trends/wp-content/uploads/sites/3/2019/04/Race-report_updated-4.29.19.pdf.

Prelow, H., Mosher, C., & Bowman, M. (2006). Perceived Racial Discrimination, Social Support, and Psychological Adjustment among African American College Students. *Journal of Black Psychology, 32*(4), 442–54.

Preuschoff, K., Quartz, S. R., & Bossaerts, P. (2008). Human insula activation reflects risk prediction errors as well as risk. *Journal of Neuroscience, 28*(11), 2745–52.

Rowen, B. & Chamberlain, L. (2022, January 13). Major Race Riots in the U.S. *Infoplease.* https://www.infoplease.com/us/history/major-race-riots-us.

Seshadri, G., & Knudson-Martin, C. (2013). How Couples Manage Interracial and Intercultural Differences: Implications for Clinical Practice. *Journal of Marital and Family Therapy, 39*(1), 43–58. doi: 10.1111/j.1752-0606.2011.00262.x.

Silvestrini, M. (2020). "It's not something I can take": The Effect of Racial Stereotypes, Beauty Standards, and Sexual Racism on Interracial Attraction. *Sexuality & Culture, 24*, 305–25.

Simon, R.W. (2002). Revisiting the Relationships among Gender, Marital Status and Mental Health. American Journal of Sociology, 107, 1065–96.

Skinner, A. L., & Hudac, C. M. (2017). 'Yuck, you disgust me!' Affective bias against interracial couples. *Journal of Experiential Social Psychology, 68*, 68–77.

Solsberry, P. W. (1994). Interracial Couples in the United State of America: Implications for Mental Health Counseling. *Journal of Mental Health Counseling, 16*(3), 304–17.

Steinbugler, A. 2014. racial divides. *Contexts, 13*(2), 32–37.

Tillman, K., & Miller, B. (2017). The role of family relationships in the psychological wellbeing of interracially dating adolescents. *Social Science Research, 65*, 240–52. https://doi.org/10.1016/j.ssresearch.2016.11.001.

Umberson, D., & Montez, J. K. (2010). Social Relationships and Health A Flashpoint for Health Policy. *Journal of Health and Social Behavior, 51*(1), 54–66.

Vaquera, E., & Kao, G. (2005). Private and Public Displays of Affection Among Interracial and Intra-Racial Adolescent Couples. *Social Science Quarterly, 86*(2), 484–509.

Waite, L. J., & Gallagher, M. (2000). *The Case for Marriage: Why Married People Are Happier, Healthier, and Better Off Financially.* New York: Doubleday.

Waite, L. J., & Lehrer, E. L. (2003). The Benefits from Marriage and Religion in the United States: A Comparative Analysis. *Population and Development Review, 29*(2), 255–75.

Williams, K., & Umberson, D. (2004). Marital Status, Marital Transitions, and Health: A Gendered Life Course Perspective. *Journal of Health and Social Behavior, 45*, 81–98.

Wong, J. S., & Penner, A. M. (2018). Better Together? Interracial Relationships and Depressive Symptoms. *Sociological Research for a Dynamic World, 4*, 1–11.

Wootson, C. R. (2016, August 16). White supremacist stabs interracial couple after seeing them kiss at bar, police say. *Washington Post*. https://www.washingtonpost.com/news/post-nation/wp/2016/08/19/white-supremacist-stabs-interracial-couple-after-seeing-them-kiss-at-bar-police-say/?utm_term=.47b31c84cd6d.

Yancey, G. (2002). Who Interracially Dates: An Examination of the Characteristics of those who have Interracially Dated. *Journal of Comparative Family Studies, 33*(2), 179–90.

Yu, Y., & Zhang, Z. (2017). Interracial Marriage and Self-Reported Health of Whites and Blacks in the United States. Population Research and Policy Review, 36(6), 851–70.

Chapter 2

Bridging Racial Groups

OVERVIEW

Few things gauge one's interest in bridging racial groups through interracial romance like the experiences a person goes through when choosing a romantic partner. The partner selection process of *assortative mating* is impacted by a number of personal and social factors that greatly influence a person's decision to choose a partner the same race as himself or herself (homogamy) or one with a different racial background (heterogamy) (Kalminj, 1998). On the surface, it may appear that the decision is fully up to the individual, but in actuality there are a variety of factors that impact a person's choice of romantic partner. The pool of available partners, social class, and physical attractiveness are just a few of the determinants people consider in the assortative mating process. For many people, the racial identity of their potential is an essential aspect of the partner selection process, especially for those who choose to cross racial lines for romance. Therefore, the purpose of this chapter is to discuss how racial identity and other factors impact the assortative mating process of the Bridge Kids and others in IRRs.

THE PARTNER SELECTION PROCESS—
ASSORTATIVE MATING

Near the turn of the twentieth century, W.E.B. DuBois wrote "the problem of the twentieth century is the problem of the color-line" (Du Bois, 1903: p. 10). In this context, DuBois' color-line is in reference to racial identity. Although the degree to which race is still a primary social problem is debatable by some, one way the color-line does continue to impact society in the twenty-first century is through the partner selection process.

The partner selection process is highly subjective, and most people form partnerships based on the principle of *assortative mating*. Assortative mating is the tendency of people to become romantically involved with someone that has similar or dissimilar genotypes (heritable genetic characteristics), phenotypes (physical characteristics), culture, religion, beliefs, education, social class, or other traits as themselves (Burke et al., 2013; Jiang, Bolnick, & Kirkpatrick, 2013). Selecting a romantic partner that has similar characteristics as oneself is referred to as "positive assortative mating" or *homogamy* (Kalminj, 1998). The preference for positive assortative mating might be best summed up by the old adage, "people like people like themselves." In contrast, partnering with someone that has dissimilar characteristics (dissortative mating) is referred to as "negative assortative mating" or *heterogamy* (Kalminj, 1998). The old adage that best reflects heterogamous relationships is "opposites attract." Nonetheless, the partner selection process is very personal and for many people, the race of their potential partner is very influential in determining whether they engage in homogamy (e.g., same-race relationships) or heterogamy (e.g., interracial relationships).

Some people that partake in heterogamy would probably argue that the color-line is still a social problem, especially if you cross that line for romance. Far too many people question the idea of finding other-race people as desirable partners and often do so with little to no consideration for the person's non-racial traits or the numerous other personal and social factors that influence who he or she selects as their mate. A person's decision to cross racial lines during the assortative mating process are shaped by the expectations and preferences of an individual's family, friends, and community as well as other determinants including the individual's gender, socioeconomic status (SES), geographic region, and use of online dating platforms. Given the importance of race in categorizing interracial relationships as such, to better understand the assortative mating of individuals like the Bridge Kids and others that are in IRRs, it is prudent to begin with an examination of the role racial identity and other factors play in the assortative mating process.

RACIAL IDENTITY

The lives people lead is intricately tied to their numerous identities such as a cultural identity, professional identity, gender identity, religious identity, and racial identity. Identity is fundamental to how we see ourselves (self-identity) as well as how others see us (social-identity). Sometimes our self-identity does not match our social identity, which can greatly affect a person's lived experiences since identities are developed and reinforced both socially and symbolically (Stryker, 1987; Stryker & Burke, 2000). This is highly relative in a racially stratified society like the United States (U.S.) where a person's identity is strongly tied to their own racial identity as well as the race of their romantic relationship (Afful, Wohlford, & Stoetling, 2015).

Racial identity in the United States has long been determined by a person's heritage, but defining race goes far beyond supposedly common-sense categories based on someone's phenotype. In the United States, "individuals are born into an already structured society" and the "social categories in which individuals place themselves [or placed by others] are parts of a structured society and exist only in relation to other contrasting categories (for example, black vs. white); each has more or less power, prestige, status, and so on" (Stets & Burke, 2000: p. 225). In this sense, in a socially stratified society like the United States, a person's racial identity is symbolic of their social status and used to denote their presumed level of power and prestige.

In the United States, the symbolic categories used for racial identification are established by the federal government's Office of Management and Budget (OMB) (census.gov 2019). Although the racial categories have changed many times over the course of U.S. history, the current census allows individuals to self-identify with one or more of the following racial groups: White; Black/African American/Negro; American Indian/Alaska Native; Asian (with specific notation for Chinese, Japanese, Filipino, Korean, Asian Indian, Vietnamese, or Other Asian), Pacific Islander (with specific notation for Native Hawaiian, Samoan, Guamanian/Chamorro, or Other Pacific Islands); or Some Other race (Pew Research Center, 2015; Pew Research Center, 2020). More recently, the ability to self-identify with two or more racial groups has subsequently led to the creation of an unofficial racial group of individuals that are socially recognized as *Multiracial*.

In addition to self-identifying with one of the broader racial groups (i.e., Asian/Pacific Islander, Black, Native American, or White), the U.S. census requires everyone to separately identify if they have Hispanic or Latino heritage (Lopez, Krogstad, & Passel 2020), resulting in the differentiation of Hispanic/Latino individuals into an ethnic group rather than a racial group. This is an important distinction because race and ethnicity are often used interchangeably, but race is used to signify a group that shares inheritable biological traits and an ethnic group are people that share a common culture, language, ancestry, and heritage (Coates, Brunsma, & Ferber, 2018; Giddens et al., 2019). Accordingly, people with Hispanic/Latino backgrounds are classified as an ethnic group whereas all others are viewed as racial groups, despite the significant pan-ethnic variation that exists within each racial group (Kim & White, 2010; Lee & Bean, 2007). For example, Jamaican, Nigerian, and American-born Blacks each have their own distinct cultures as do Chinese, Japanese, Filipinos, Laotians, and American-born Asians. The same is also true among Native Americans (e.g., Cherokee, Sioux, Apache,

Iroquois) as well as Whites (e.g., Irish, Italian, French, Russian). Given that all recognized racial groups have a degree of pan-ethnic variation like those with Hispanic/Latino heritage, I respectfully use the term "race" in reference to those individuals that identify as Asian, Black, Hispanic, Native American, White, and Multiracial.

When considering the partner selection process, racial identity is a highly influential factor that was a long used as part of the criteria for who could and could not legally engage in romantic relationships. For most of American history, *anti-miscegenation* laws were enforced in many parts of the country that prevented people with different racial identities, particularly Whites and Nonwhites, from engaging in romantic relationships or marriage (Browning, 1951; Gordon, 1964). Even in parts of the country where interracial romance was legal, it was highly frowned upon and considered socially taboo (Browning, 1951). As a result, labeling one's romantic *relationship type* as either a same race relationship (SRR) or an interracial relationship (IRR) as well as the specific racial identity of each partner constituting the romantic *couple's racial composition* (e.g., Asian-Black, Hispanic-White, Native American-White) have almost always been notable issues in the partner selection process.

Like the racial identity of an individual, the racial identity of a romantic couple can seriously affect the lived experiences of both partners. Although IRRs are now much more socially acceptable than in the past, they have always been stigmatized and faced a level of social opposition (Browning, 1954; Gordon, 1964; McCarthy, 2021). Consequently, interracial couples are often looked at and treated differently than those in SRRs. For example, in 2009, a justice of the peace blatantly refused to perform a wedding ceremony for a Black-White couple in the state of Louisiana because he didn't "do interracial weddings" mainly out of "concern for the children" (CNN.com, 2009), and after yelling a racial slur, a self-proclaimed white supremacist stabbed a Black man and his White girlfriend in Olympia, Washington after seeing them kiss in public (Wootson, 2016). For these and other interracial couples, the stress and emotional strain associated with such traumatic experiences, or wondering if one's self or one's partner will also be victimized, probably contribute to the greater anxiety, psychological distress and depressive symptomatology reported by people in IRRs compared to those in SRRs (Barr & Simon, 2014; Bratter & Eschbach, 2006; Tillman & Miller, 2017; Wong & Penner, 2018). Thus, it appears that relationship type *does* matter because the stigma associated with interracial romance can adversely affect the lived experiences of those in IRRs by exposing them to social stressors persons in SRRs do not have to deal with.

SOCIAL CONSTRUCTION OF RACE

I believe it needs to be clearly understood that stigmatizing and unfairly treating people in IRRs based on the presumption that people with different racial identities are inherently different is unwarranted and unjust behavior. The reason being is that researchers use contemporary studies from the natural and social sciences that presents a plethora of empirical evidence demonstrating that race is not biological but rather a socially constructed concept. This rationale is supported by the *social constructivism theory*, which suggests that human life and our understanding of the world is largely attributed to social and interpersonal factors like social groups and institutions that are constructed by people (Detel, 2015; Galbin ,2014). People then perceive these social constructs to be real and accept them as part of the reality of their lives (Amineh & Asl, 2015). Race is therefore a social construct because it is "an idea that has been created and accepted by the people in a society" (Merrimamwebster.com, 2020). *Symbolic interactionist theory* contends that social constructs, such as race, derive their meanings from social interactions (Aksan et al., 2009). Through our interactions with others, generation after generation, people learn that race and racial groups are symbolic of one's positionality in a socially stratified society. It is in this way that the meaning of constructs like race and interracial couples are socially constructed.

Following this same logic, a similar argument can be used to demonstrate the geographic regions the U.S. census uses for its racial categories (i.e., Africa, America, Asia, Europe, and Latin America) are also socially constructed. As clearly depicted when viewing images of the Earth taken from outer space, Africa, Europe, and Asia are all connected as one gigantic land mass, as are the Americas. There are absolutely no distinct delineations, other than the oceans and other bodies of water, that separate where one continental land mass, country, state, or province ends, and another begins. Thus, geographic borders, like racial identities, are man-made divisions that have shifted over time and only have real meanings because people accept them as real.

Human populations are not static either since people have almost always migrated across socially constructed borders and in doing so, they often merged their cultures and genetics by means of assortative mating and reproduction. The incessant migration and blending of human cultures and families from different areas of the world for millennia makes the idea of establishing clearly distinct boundaries between "racial" groups highly implausible if not outright impossible. Rather, racial identity is a function of one's color and culture.

Even when taking geography into account, some people argue that race is real because people from different geographic regions tend to have different skin tones and other phenotype differences. However, this argument has been disproven by research showing the deoxyribonucleic acid (DNA)—genetically heritable material—of any two human beings are 99.9 percent identical (Crow, 2002; Genome.gov, 2019). Moreover, of the 0.1 percent variation in human DNA, there is greater genetic variation within the populations of Africa, Asian, and Europe people (85–90 percent) then the 10–15 percent variation between them (AAA, 1998; Genome.gov, 2019; Jorde & Wooding, 2004). That is to say, most genetic variation (about 90 percent) is found within a single continental group but there are only slight differences (about 10 percent) among the broader human population. This means Whites (Europeans) are genetically more like Blacks (Africans) or Asians than to other Whites. Therefore, regardless of geography, our skin tone and other phenotype differences only partially make up the tiny 0.1 percent genetic variations found between us (Jorde & Wooding 2004) because no matter how people divide the Earth or the racial categories created, we are genetically far more alike than different.

Regarding the genetics of race, the most thorough and definitive findings of any genetic study to date come from the Human Genome Project (HGP). The HGP was a monumental and extensive collaboration of an international team of scientists (including but not limited to biologists, computer programmers, geneticists, and physicians) from the United States, France, China, Germany, the United Kingdom, and Japan that was funded by the National Institute of Health (NIH) and the Department of Energy. Headed by James Watson (co-winner of the 1962 Nobel Prize in Philosophy of Medicine for the discovery of the double-helical structure of DNA), the HGP ran from 1990 to 2003 and sequenced the three billion pairs of nucleotides that form a complete set of DNA molecules found in human chromosomes. The findings of this extensive collaboration revealed that there are no genetic markers that distinguish any clear and distinct racial groups among humans (Genome.gov, 2019). Simply put, people need to be informed and accept the fact that the ideas of race and racially superior or inferior groups are nonsensical if the person who discovered DNA says no gene for race exists.

Even the Office of Management and Budget (OMB) acknowledges the racial classifications used by the U.S. government "generally reflect a social definition of race recognized in this country and [are] not an attempt to define race biologically, anthropologically, or genetically" (Census.gov, 2019). This statement staunchly aligns with the science that finds race is neither genetic nor immutable, but rather a set of socially constructed categories that have long been accepted by many people in our society. Given how deeply these ideas of racial division have been incorporated into our society, the tenets of the Thomas Theorem imply that although modern science clearly shows that race is not real, if people view race as real then its consequences will also be real (Bornmann & Marx, 2020). Thus, while science and even the U.S. government recognizes that race is not biologically "real," it is nonetheless socially real in its consequence. By extension, the idea of "interracial relationships" is not real either and the disdain some feel for mixed-race partnerships is founded on the false belief in racial differences, but there are still real consequences on the lived experiences and well-being of those in such relationships that also influence some people's decision on whether to cross racial lines when selecting a romantic partner.

SKIN TONE

The racial identity of individuals and interracial couples is often based on each person's skin tone. For some people, their skin tone is perhaps equally important as their racial self-identity in terms of being a salient characteristic that influences their assortative mating process. Labels such as "Black" and "White" clearly indicate that a darker complexion is associated with having African ancestry and a fair skin tone signifies Caucasian descent (Hall 2019). Since many Americans oppose interracial romance and individuals in IRRs are often exposed to discrimination (Steinbugler, 2014; Yancey, 2007), people may be more likely to choose a partner with a similar skin tone as themselves to avoid being socially stigmatized for being in an IRR. Accordingly, skin tone is an important trait in partner selection because it is often used as a proxy for a person's race and their social status.

In the United States, the fair skin of White people is often promoted and idolized, leading to the perception that fair skin is linked to beauty and dark skin is associated with unattractiveness (Arif, 2004; Bauman, 2008). Concerning romantic attraction, most Americans seem to have a clear preference for lighter and tanned skin and are much less attracted to Black and very light skin (Aoki, 2002; Frisby, 2006). For instance, a young adult male that racially identifies as Indian stated he is more attracted to White women than any other racial identity "because of how things are portrayed in popular culture. When you look around, you see a lot of White people and light-skinned Black people, certain types of looks and things like that. So, when you see that, you're more familiar with it, and I feel like you're more attracted to things that you're familiar with" (Silvestrini, 2020; p. 317). Accordingly, regardless of one's own skin tone or racial identity, people with fairer skin tones tend to be seen as a more desirable partner because they are perceived as being more physically attractive by many potential mates (Marway, 2018).

Variations in skin tone are also linked to how people are perceived and treated by others (Craig 2002; Rowland and Burris 2017). This is particularly important in a society where those with fair skin tones, like many White people, are typically engendered with special privileges. This *white privilege*, the "acknowledged and unearned assets that benefit Whites in their everyday lives" (Giddens et al., 2019: p. 298), helps make White individuals more desirable partners. Yet, there is extraordinary variation in skin tone across the color spectrum (Blum, 2002), as skin color varies with genetic ancestry (Charles, 2003). People that identify as Asian, Black, Hispanic, and Native American have wide-ranging skin complexions from very fair to very dark (Deng & Xu, 2018; Reece, 2019). The varied skin tones of many of these individuals make it difficult to categorize them into one mutually exclusive racial group, thereby giving many Nonwhite people a *racially ambiguous* appearance. As such, people that appear White, racial minorities whose skin complexions are White-passing, or those that appear racially ambiguous, are likely to be viewed as more desirable partners.

GENDER

Women and men often find different traits desirable in a partner, so gender is another key characteristic in the assortative mating process. Given the subjectivity of the partner selection process and near countless reasons men and women have for choosing their romantic partners, I will primarily focus on gender differences in couples' racial compositions. In terms of interracial partnerships, the average age for newlywed men and women is about 35 and 32, respectively, and the age for intermarried men is 34 and women 32. The mean age difference between intermarried husbands and wives is about 2.8 years, which is consistent across White-Nonwhite partnerships, with the smallest difference for pairings between Hispanic husbands with White wives (2.1 years), and the largest between White husbands with Asian wives (4.6 years) (Wang, 2012).

In general, men and women are near equally likely to be in an IRR. For example, as presented in Figure 2.1, data from the Pew Research Center presented in the work of Livingston and Brown (2017) shows that, although women and men are equally likely to be in interracial relationships, the prevalence of interracial romance varies by the intersection of race and gender. For instance, 21 percent of Asian men, 36 percent of Asian women, 24 percent of Black men, 12 percent of Black women, 26 percent of Hispanic men, 28 percent of Hispanic women, 12 percent of White men, and 10 percent of White women interracially married as newlyweds in 2015 (Pew Research Center, 2017). Thus, proportionally, there are a range of gender differences in interracial involvement within racial groups, with the most pronounced difference in prevalence being among Asian and Black men and women.

% of U.S. newlyweds who are intermarried

■ Men ■ Women

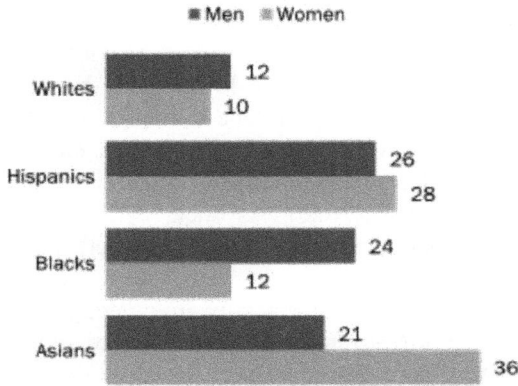

Whites 12 / 10
Hispanics 26 / 28
Blacks 24 / 12
Asians 21 / 36

Note: Whites, blacks and Asians include only non-Hispanics.
Hispanics are of any race. Asians include Pacific Islanders.
Source: Pew Research Center analysis of 2014-2015 American
Community Survey (IPUMS).
"Intermarriage in the U.S. 50 Years After Loving v. Virginia"

PEW RESEARCH CENTER

Figure 2.1. Race and Gender Differences in Newlyweds Who Are Intermarried. "U.S. Approval of Interracial Marriage at New High of 94%." Pew Research Center, Washington, D.C. (September 10, 2021) https://news.gallup.com/poll/354638/approval -interracialmarriage-new-high.aspx?version=print

The most significant gender differences are seen when looking at who men and women partner with when they cross racial lines for romance. These dissimilarities are much more pronounced among Whites, as nearly half of intermarried White men and women have Hispanic spouses. However, White men are more likely to have a wife who is Asian (27 percent) than Black (7 percent) whereas White women are more likely to have a husband who is Black (20 percent) than Asian (9 percent) (Passel et al., 2010). A similar pattern is also found among interracially involved teenagers (Kreager, 2008; Vaquera & Kao, 2005). Therefore, when looking at *who* men and women cross racial lines for, it is clear that regardless of race or gender, most interracially involved racial minorities have White partners and interracial relations between two minorities is much less common.

SOCIOECONOMIC STATUS (SES)

Two personal traits most men and women find desirable in a partner are high incomes and educational attainment, which are both measures of a person's socioeconomic status (SES). SES represents the social and economic background of an individual or household assessed by factors such as wealth, prestige, poverty, occupation, income, and educational attainment (Villalba, 2014). There is meaningful variation in SES across race however, as Black, and Hispanic persons generally have lower SES than Whites and Asians (Giddens et al., 2019; Wang, 2012). Due to their lower average SES, racial minorities are less likely to be viewed as an acceptable partner, particularly by some White individuals or the members of their broader social networks (Burnett, 2014, Silvestrini, 2020). As such, SES is a characteristic that tends to strongly influence a person's decision whether to cross racial lines for romance.

For those that do become interracially involved, the median household income of racial minorities intermarried to a White spouse is significantly greater than those in same-race marriages. Research by Wang (2012) shows the combined income of newlywed interracial couples is $69,900 compared to $67,400 for same-race couples. More specifically, as shown in Table 2.1, Wang (2012) finds that the income for the average White-White household that was newlywed between 2008 and 2010 is $60,000, whereas the income for White-Asian households is about $71,000, Asian-Asian $62,000, Hispanic-White $58,000, Hispanic-Hispanic $35,600, Black-White $53,000, and Black-Black $47,700.

The observed differences in household income may at least be partially due to differences in educational attainment, as higher educational attainment is strongly associated with higher earning occupations (Wolla & Sullivan, 2017). In terms of both partners being college educated, the overall findings by Wang (2012), which are also presented in Table 2.1, point to the importance of educational attainment in the interracial partner selection process as Blacks and Hispanics that are intermarried to a White spouse have relatively higher educational attainment than those in same-race marriages. This is particularly true for Black men and Hispanic men. This also suggests that White men appear to find minority women as desirable partners if they are college educated, which further strengthens the argument that people find educated partners attractive (sapiophile) above and beyond their racial identity. Taken together, the data points to a *partner premium* for higher SES racial minorities who tend to be more structurally assimilated into larger groups and social institutions that provide them with greater opportunities for intergroup interactions that make them viewed as desirable partners by White persons.

Table 2.1. Household Income and Education of Newlywed Couples. Data used to create the graph was retrieved from "The Rise of Intermarriage." Pew Research Center, Washington, D.C. (February 16, 2012). https://www.pewresearch.org/social-trends /2012/02/16/the-rise-of-interrmarriage/

	Household Income	Both College Educated
Race and Gender		
AM-AF	$62,000	62%
AM-WF	$72,000	61%
AF-WM	$71,000	60%
BM-BF	$48,000	18%
BM-WF	$53,000	20%
BF-WM	$61,000	31%
HM-HF	$36,000	10%
HM-WF	$53,000	23%
HF-WM	$61,000	33%
WM-WF	$60,000	32%

Note: AM=Asian Male, AF= Asian Female BM=Black Male, BF=Black Female HM=Hispanic Male, HF=Hispanic Female WM=White Male, WF=White Female

Note: dollars rounded to nearest thousand.

partner premium for higher SES racial minorities who tend to be more structurally assimilated into larger groups and social institutions that provide them with greater opportunities for intergroup interactions that make them viewed as desirable partners by White persons.

GEOGRAPHY

Apart from individual-level attributes like race, gender, SES, and other characteristics a person deems desirable in a partner, interracial romantic involvement is also profoundly affected by geographic proximity. While the decline of *de jure* segregation (mandated by law) has meant that people of differing racial groups hypothetically have more opportunities to interact with one another on a social level, geographic proximity to other-race groups remains limited due to the *de facto* segregation (due to social differences) that is still prevalent across much of the United States. In many parts of the United States, racially segregated people have fewer real opportunities to interact, and develop intimate relationships, with others from different racial groups then their own. It is therefore plausible that the racial diversity of a person's community and geographic region effect their ability to have meaningful mixed-race social interactions and form interracial romantic relationships.

For instance, intermarriage is most prevalent in cities like Honolulu, Hawaii; Las Vegas, Nevada; and Santa Barbara, California, where there are high proportions of both Whites and racial minorities. On the other hand, IRRs are least common in cities like Youngstown, Ohio; Ashville, North Carolina; and Jackson, Mississippi, where there are far fewer minorities and much less racial diversity (Livingston & Brown 2017; Pew Research Center 2017). When focusing on the broader geographic regions, it may be surprising to some that the highest proportion of intermarried couples is in the Southern region of the United States (36 percent) followed by the West (35.1 percent), Midwest (16.1 percent), and the lowest is in the Northeast (12.8 percent) (Wang, 2012), but follows the pattern of racial propinquity as the South and West are the more racially diverse regions in the country (Frey, 2019). This is particularly interesting since people in the South and Midwest are less accepting of IRRs and more likely to view them as bad for society than those in the West (Pew Research Center, 2017). The data seems to indicate that when given the opportunity, people are willing to form IRRs, even in areas where such relationships are frowned upon.

The juxtaposition between the high prevalence of IRRs in areas with high levels of social disapproval makes it more complex to link interracial involvement to attitudes on large regional scales. Geographically, large regions like the South or Northeast have vast rural areas where attitudes of IRRs as good for society are substantially lower (24 percent) than in urban areas (45 percent) (Pew Research Center, 2017). Cities also tend to be more racially diverse than rural areas, which is likely a factor contributing to the higher prevalence of interracial couples in urban areas (Miller et al., 2021; Pew Research Center, 2017). It therefore appears that interracial partner selection is associated with both the racial diversity *and* people's attitudes towards interracial romance in the specific geographic locations a person lives.

ONLINE DATING

One way more and more people are dealing with the issue of geographically limited partner selection pools is through online dating. The use of online dating websites and cellular phone dating applications (apps) is a contemporary strategy millions of people use to bridge races and spaces for their partner selection processes. Nearly one-third of U.S. adults have used an online dating site or an app, half of which are young adults ages 18–29, like the Bridge Kids (Pew Research Center, 2020). The emergence of websites like Match.com and eharmony.com have increased the opportunities of the Bridge Kids and other people searching for romantic partners to date and specify the characteristics they like and dislike in a mate, including their race.

Online daters can indicate the extent race plays a role in their partner selection by indicating in their profiles: 1) the race(s) of people in which they are not interested; 2) if they are open to people of any race; and 3) the race(s) of the people they are interested in, which could be either a same-race or interracial partner (Buggs, 2017; Hwang, 2013). As an Asian young man pointed out, "On Grindr, . . . [p]eople will put in their bios what race they're into or not into, like say things like 'No Asians' or 'No Blacks'" (Silvestrini, 2020; p. 320). There are also a number of dating sites such as asiandating.com (Asians), blackpeoplemeet.com (Blacks), amigos.com (Hispanics/Latinos), and meetnativeamericans.com (Native Americans) that cater to people looking to meet a partner with a specific racial identity. The diversity of these online dating platforms gives people numerous options to structure and engage in their search, which serve as powerful tools in the interracial partner selection process.

The work of Mendelsohn and colleagues (2014) found the profiles of most online users on a popular dating site clearly expressed a preference for a same-race partner, notably White users made this designation more than Blacks, women more than men, and older persons more than young. Also, while the preference for only being in an IRR was only 2 percent for White users and 6 percent for Blacks, only 3 percent of contacts initiated by Whites were to Blacks whereas 37 percent of contacts initiated by Blacks were to Whites. In sum, the findings by Mendelsohn and colleagues (2014) indicate that, for most people using the more popular dating sites, race is in fact a salient characteristic they consider in the partner selection process. Further, albeit the majority of online users on the popular dating site prefer same-race partners, there is still clearly a pool of people that prefer to engage in interracial relationships and an even larger group who are at least willing to cross racial lines for romance.

Appropriately, not only do online dating sites give people greater accessibility to form same-race partnerships, but they also serve as broader forums for those searching for, or open to, interracial involvement. In fact, there are several websites including swirlr.com, interracialpeoplemeet.com, and interracialcupid.com that are intended for people who are specifically interested in interracial relationships. It is also probable that an analysis of the users on these specialized dating sites have a much higher desire for interracial romance than the popular site analyzed by Mendelsohn and colleagues (2014). In this sense, online dating may be one way for some individuals to actively seek out partners from other racial groups to engage in interracial romance without the stigmatization or backlash from those that disapprove of interracial romance, or due to the lack of racial diversity in their geographic location. Such a strategy may protect the mental health of those that form IRRs through online forums by buffering their psychological well-being from the adverse effects of being exposed to stigma and discrimination from those that might oppose their relationship during the partner selection process.

A study by Hergovich and Ortega (2018) noted that, although the number of interracial marriages has steadily increased since 1970, the rate of this increase becomes much higher around 2006 when well-known online platforms like OKCupid became popularized. After analyzing the data, the researchers conclude that online dating is actually leading to more interracial marriages. These findings can probably be extrapolated to other less formal types of relationships with the assumption that the use of online dating websites contribute to greater interracial hookups, interracial dating, and interracial cohabitation, as well as intermarriage and Multiracial family formation. This is probably especially true for young adults like the Bridge Kids that are most likely to use online dating sites and apps (Pew Research Center, 2020), suggesting the trend of increasing rates of interracial involvement through online forums will continue into the foreseeable future.

CONCLUSION

It is clear that, for some people, considering the race and skin tone of their partner is a vital aspect of their partner selection process. If more people were made aware that race is a nonsensical social construct, especially when they are young, racial identity would undoubtedly have less influence on the partner selection process. Less racial division, in turn, is likely to contribute to greater social cohesion in our society. As noted by Hergovich and Ortega (2018) "a few interracial links can lead to a significant increase in the racial integration of our societies, and leads to optimistic views on the role that dating platforms can play in modern civilizations" (p. 22). They go on to deduce that the number of interracial marriages will increase as online dating becomes even more popular. Given that interracial couples serve as a bridge between multiple racial groups as well as an indicator of a society's racial ideology (Gordon, 1964; Joyner & Kao, 2005; Miller, 2014), the racial beliefs and assortative mating patterns of the Bridge Kids can be seen as a lens for predicting how they will shape future ideas of race and race relations.

REFERENCES

Afful, S. E., Wohlford, C., & Stoelting, S. M. (2015). Beyond 'Difference': Examining the Process and Flexibility of Racial Identity in Interracial Marriages. *Journal of Social Issues, 71*(4), 659–74.

Aksan, N., Kisac, B., Aydin, M., & Demirbuken, S. (2009). Symbolic interaction theory. *Procedia Social and Behavioral Sciences, 1*, 902–04.

American Anthropological Association. (1998). *American Anthropological Association Statement on Race.* https://www.americananthro.org/ConnectWithAAA/Content.aspx?ItemNumber=2583.

Amineh, R. J., & Asl, H. D. (2015). Review of Constructivism and Social Constructivism. *Journal of Social Sciences, Literature, and Languages, 1*, 9–16.

Aoki, K. (2001). Sexual selection as a cause of human skin colour variation: Darwin's hypothesis revisited. *Annals of Human Biology, 29*(6), 589–608.

Arif, H. (2004). Woman's body as a color measuring text: A signification of Bengali culture. *Semiotica, 150*(1/4), 579–95.

Barr, A. B. & Simons, R. L. (2014). A Dyadic Analysis of Relationships and Health: Does Couple-level Context Condition Partner Effects?" *Journal of Family Psychology, 28*(4), 448–59.

Baumann, S. (2008). The moral underpinnings of beauty: A meaning-based explanation for light and dark complexions in advertising. *Poetics, 36*(1), 2–23.

Blum, L. (2002). *I'm not a racist, but . . . : The moral quandary of race*. Cornell University Press.

Bornmann, L., & Marx, W. (2020). Thomas theorem in research evaluation. *Scientometrics, 123*, 553–55. https://doi.org/10.1007/s11192-020-03389-6.

Bratter, J., & Eschbach, K. (2006). What about the couple? Interracial marriage and psychological distress. *Social Science Research, 35*, 1025–47.

Browning, J. (1951). Anti-Miscegenation Laws in the United States. 1 *Duke Bar Journal*, 26–41. http://scholarship.law.duke.edu/dlj/vol1/iss1/3.

Burke, D., Nolan, C., Hayward, W. G., Russell, R., & Sulikowski, D. (2013). Is There an Own-Race Preference in Attractiveness?. *Evolutionary Psychology, 11*(4), 855–72.

Burnett, Erika. 2014. *Interracial Relationships and Social Exchange Theory*. https://erikaburnettblog.wordpress.com/2014/05/04/interracial-relationships-and-social-exchange-theory/.

Charles, C. A. D. (2003). Skin bleaching, self-hate, and black identity in Jamaica. *Journal of Black Studies, 33*(6), 711–28.

CNN.com. (2009, November 3). *Louisiana justice who refused interracial marriage resigns. CNN.* http://www.cnn.com/2009/US/11/03/louisiana.interracial.marriage/index.html.

Coates, R. D., Brunsma, D. L., & Ferber, A. L. (2018). *The matrix of race: social construction, intersectionality, and inequality*. Sage Publications.

Craig, M. L. (2002). *Ain't I a beauty queen? Black women, beauty, and the politics of race*. Oxford University Press.

Crow, J. F. (2002). Unequal by nature: a geneticist's perspective on human differences. Daedelus: *Journal of the American Academy of Arts & Sciences, Winter*, 81–88.

Deng, L. & Xu, S. (2018). Adaptation of human skin color in various populations. *Hereditas, 155*(1), 1–12. https://www.ncbi.nlm.nih.gov/pmc/articles/PMC5502412/.

Detel, W. (2015). *Social Constructivism. International Encyclopedia of the Social & Behavioral Sciences* (Second Edition), 228–34.

Du Bois, W. E. B. (1903). *The Souls of Black Folk*. A.C. McClurg & Co.

Frey, W. H. (2019). *Six maps that reveal America's expanding racial diversity*. https://www.brookings.edu/research/americas-racial-diversity-in-six-maps/.

Frisby, C. M. (2006). Shades of beauty: examining the relationship of skin color to perceptions of physical attractiveness. *Facial Plastic Surgery, 22*(3), 175–79.

Galbin, A. (2014). An Introduction to Social Constructionism. *Social Research Reports, 26,* 82–92. https://www.researchreports.ro/an-introduction-to-social-constructionism.

Giddens A., Mitchell, D., Richard, A., & Carr, D. (Eds.). (2019). *Essentials of Sociology, 7th edition.* W. W. Norton and Company Publications.

Gordon, M. (1964). *Assimilation in American Life: The Role of Race, Religion, and National Origin.* Oxford University Press.

Hall, R. (2019). From race to melanin matters: The mathematics of skin color. *LaPeaulogie, 3.* http://lapeaulogie.fr/from-race-to-melanin-matters-the-mathematics-of-skin-color/.

Hergovich, P., & Ortega, J. (2018). The Strength of Absent Ties: Social Integration via Online Dating. *SSRN.* https://papers.ssrn.com/sol3/papers.cfm?abstract_id=3044766.

Human Genome Project. (2019). *The Human Genome Project. National Human Genome Research Institute.* https://www.genome.gov/human-genome-project.

Hwang, C. (2013). Who are People Willing to Date? Ethnic and Gender Patterns on Online Dating. *Race and Social Problems, 5*(1), 28–40.

Jiang, Y, Bolnick, D. I. & Kirkpatrick, M. (2013). Assortative Mating in Animals. *The American Naturalist, 181*(6), E125–E138.

Jorde, L. B., & Wooding, S. P. (2004). Genetic variation, classification and 'race.' *Nature genetics, 36*(11), 528–33.

Joyner, K., & Kao, G. (2005). Interracial Relationships and the Transition to Adulthood. *American Sociological Review, 70,* 563–81.

Kalmijn, M. (1998). Intermarriage and Homogamy: Causes, Patterns, Trends. *Annual Review of Sociology, 24,* 395–421.

Kim, A. H., & White, M. J. (2010). Panethnicity, ethnic diversity, and residential segregation. *American Journal of Sociology, 115*(5), 1558–96.

Kreager, D. (2008). Guarded Borders: Adolescent Interracial Romance and Peer Trouble at School. *Social Forces, 87*(2), 887–910.

Lee, J., & Bean, F. D. (2007). Reinventing the Color Line: Immigration and America's New Racial/Ethnic Divide. *Social Forces, 86*(2), 561–86.

Livingston, G., & Brown, A. (2017, May 18). Intermarriage in the U.S. 50 Years After Loving v. Virginia. *Pew Research Center.* https://www.pewresearch.org/social-trends/2017/05/18/intermarriage-in-the-u-s-50-years-after-loving-v-virginia/.

Lopez, M. H., Krogstad, J. M., & Passel, J. S. (2020, September 15). Who is Hispanic?. *Pew Research Center.* https://www.pewresearch.org/fact-tank/2020/09/15/who-is-hispanic/.

Marway, H. (2018). Should We Genetically Select for the Beauty Norm of Fair Skin?. *Health Care Anal, 26,* 246–68.

McCarthy, J. (2021, September 10). U.S. Approval of Interracial Marriage at New High of 94%. *Gallup.* https://news.gallup.com/poll/354638/approval-interracial-marriage-new-high.aspx?version=print.

Mendelsohn, G. A., Taylor, L. S., Fiore, A. T., Ceshire, C. (2014). Black/White Dating Online: Interracial Courtship in the 21st Century. *Psychology of Popular Media Culture, 3*(1), 2–18.

Merriam-Webeter Dictionary. (2020). *Social Construct.* https://www.merriam-webster .com/dictionary/social%20construct.

Miller, B. (2014). What are the odds: An examination of adolescent interracial romance and risk for depression. *Youth & Society, 49*(2), 180–202.

Miller, B., Catalina, S., Rocks, S., & Tillman, K. (2021). It Is Your Decision to Date Interracially: The Influence of Family Approval on the Likelihood of Interracial/Interethnic Dating. *Journal of Family Issues, 43*(2), 443–66.

Passel, J., Wang, W., & Taylor, P. (2010, June 4). Marrying Out: One-in-Seven New U.S. Marriages is Interracial or Interethnic. *Pew Research Center's Social & Demographic Trends Project.* https://www.pewresearch.org/social-trends/2010/06 /04/marrying-out/.

Pew Research Center (2012). "The Rise of Intermarriage." Pew Research Center, Washington, D.C. (February 16, 2012). https://www.pewresearch.org/social-trends /2012/02/16/the-rise-of-intermarriage/.

Pew Research Center. (2015). *Multiracial in America: Proud, Diverse and Growing in Numbers.* https://www.pewresearch.org/social-trends/2015/06/11/multiracial-in -america/.

Pew Research Center. (2017). *Intermarriage in the U.S. 50 Years After Loving v. Virginia.* http://www.pewsocialtrends.org/2017/05/18/intermarriage-in-the-u-s-50 -years-after-loving-v-virginia/.

Pew Research Center. (2020). *What Census Calls Us.* https://www.pewresearch.org/ interactives/what-census-calls-us/.

Pew Research Center. (2020). *The Virtues and Downsides of Online Dating.* https: //www.pewresearch.org/internet/2020/02/06/the-virtues-and-downsides-of-online -dating/.

Pew Research Center. (2021). "U.S. Approval of Interracial Marriage at New High of 94%." Pew Research Center, Washington, D.C. (September 10, 2021). https://news.gallup.com/poll/354638/approval-interracialmarriage-new-high.aspx ?version=print.

Reece, R. L. (2019). Coloring Racial Fluidity: How Skin Tone Shaoes Multiracial Adolescents' Racial Identity Changes. *Race and Social Problems, 11*, 290–98.

Rowland, H. M., & Burriss, R. P. (2017) Human colour in mate choice and competi-tion. *Philosophical Transactions of the Royal Society, B, 372,* 1–11.

Silvestrini, M. (2020). "It's not something I can take": The Effect of Racial Stereotypes, Beauty Standards, and Sexual Racism on Interracial Attraction. *Sexuality & Culture, 24,* 305–25.

Steinbugler, A. (2014). racial divides. *Contexts, 13*(2), 32–37.

Stets, J. E., & Burke, P. J. (2000). Identity theory and social identity theory. Social Psychology Quarterly, 63(3), 224–37. https://doi.org/10.2307/2695870.

Stryker, S. (1987). The Vitalization of Symbolic Interaction. *Social Psychology Quarterly, 50*(1), 83–94.

Stryker, S., & Burke, P.J. (2000). The Past, Present, and Future of an Identity Theory. *Social Psychology Quarterly, 63*(4), 284–97.

Tillman, K., & Miller, B. (2017). The role of family relationships in the psychological wellbeing of interracially dating adolescents. *Social Science Research, 65*, 240–52.

United States Census Bureau. (2019). *Race*. https://www.census.gov/topics/population /race/about.html.

Vaquera, E., & Kao, G. (2005). Private and Public Displays of Affection Among Interracial and Intra-Racial Adolescent Couples. *Social Science Quarterly, 86*(2), 484–509.

Villalba C.M.H. (2014) Socioeconomic Status (SES). In: Michalos A.C. (eds) *Encyclopedia of Quality of Life and Well-Being Research*. Springer, Dordrecht. https://doi.org/10.1007/978-94-007-0753-5_2805.

Wang, W. (2012, February 16). The Rise of Intermarriage: Rates, Characteristics Vary by Race and Gender. *Pew Research Center*. https://www.pewresearch.org /social- trends/2012/02/16/the-rise-of-intermarriage/.

Wolla, S. A., & Sullivan, J. (2017). Education, Income, and Wealth. Page One Economics. https://research.stlouisfed.org/publications/page1-econ/2017/01/03/ education-income-and-wealth/.

Wong, J. S., & Penner, A. M. (2018). Better Together? Interracial Relationships and Depressive Symptoms. *Sociological Research for a Dynamic World, 4*, 1–11.

Wootson, C. R. (2016, August 16). White supremacist stabs interracial couple after seeing them kiss at bar, police say. *Washington Post*. https://www.washingtonpost .com/news/post-nation/wp/2016/08/19/white-supremacist-stabs-interracial-couple -after-seeing-them-kiss-at-bar-police-say/?utm_term=.47b31c84cd6d.

Yancey, G. (2007). Experiencing Racism: Differences in the Experiences of Whites Married to Blacks and Non-Black Racial Minorities. *Journal of Comparative Family Studies, 38*(2), 197–213.

Chapter 3

Bridging Health and Well-Being

CHAPTER OVERVIEW

Health and well-being are fundamentally important to most people, and having a healthy society is a major public health issue in the United States. Accordingly, Americans spent over $4 trillion on healthcare in 2020, or about $12,500 per person, toward his or her health and well-being (cms.gov, 2021). Health outcomes are strongly linked to a person's romantic relationship status, so examining the health of romantically partnered individuals has become an essential public health issue. Which means that in addition to the attributes of the individual, it is also essential to account for the characteristics of a person's partner to gain a broader understanding of the underlying determinants of health outcomes. Furthermore, as the number of people romantically involved in interracial relationships (IRRs) continues to increase (Pew Research Center, 2017), it is now more salient than ever to include this population in the romantic disparities in health literature.

After selecting their romantic partner through the assortative mating process, most people in interracial relationships (IRRs) desire to live a long and happy life with their partners just like those in same-race relationships (SRRs). However, there are a variety of social stressors like discrimination and racism directly related to their relationship that people in IRRs must often endure that those in SRRs do not. Due to the deleterious effects that social strain and stress exposure can have on an individual's life and well-being, people in IRRs generally report having poorer health than those in SRRs (Barr & Simons, 2015; Bratter & Eschbach, 2006; Miller, 2014; Tillman & Miller, 2017; Wong & Penner, 2018). Nonetheless, relatively little is known about the health and well-being of those in IRRs or why it differs from those in SRRs. As such, the purpose of this chapter is to use the sociological study of stress perspective (Pearlin, 1989; Pearlin et al., 1981) to explore the determinants and pathways that affect the health of the Bridge Kids and others in IRRs.

INTERRACIAL ROMANCE AND HEALTH

Good health and well-being are fundamental to most people living a happy and healthy life, but understanding the countless determinants that impact a person's well-being can be quite complex. One factor that is consistently shown to be a strong predictor of a person's health is their romantic relationship status (e.g., married vs. unmarried), which shows romantically involved adults generally have better health than their unmarried counterparts (Ramanzankhani, Azizi, & Hadaegh, 2019; Robards et al., 2012). Moreover, there is a *spousal health advantage*, whereby married persons tend to live happier (Khodarahimi, 2015) and longer lives (Jia & Lubetkin, 2020) than their non-married counterparts. Thus, romantic involvement appears to be one factor that is strongly related to a person's health.

Relationships do not occur in a vacuum, however, but rather are bi-directional social relationships. This means romantic partnerships are reciprocal relationships whereby the actions, experiences, and resources of each person can affect different many aspects of their own physical, psychological, and social well-being (Kansky, 2018; Kiecolt-Glaser & Wilson, 2017), as well as their partner's. Moreover, health outcomes are associated with a number of factors including genetics, health behaviors, social environment, stress exposure, and the availability of coping resources (Barr, 2019; Genome.gov, 2021; Pearlin, 1989). Therefore, when considering the lives and well-being of people in romantic relationships, it is also important to account for the impact one's partner has on their health.

Despite the fact that interracial partnerships are becoming increasingly common in American society (Qian & Lichter, 2011; Wang, 2012) what we know about the health of those in IRRs has lagged because researchers have primarily focused on the health of people in same-race relationships (SRRs). It is especially important to address this gap in the literature because we know there are significant racial disparities in health (Marquez-Velarde, Jones, & Keith, 2020; Miller & Taylor, 2012; Williams, Lawrence, & Davis, 2019), which is particularly salient for individuals in interracial relationships (IRRs). Given the history of anti-miscegenation laws and norms against interracial marriage (Herman & Campbell, 2012; Sohoni, 2007), elevated stress burdens of racial minorities that may spill over across partners (Clavel, Cutrona, & Russell, 2017; LeBlanc, Frost, & Wight, 2015), and general opposition to interracial romance (Jones, 2005; Pew Research Center, 2017), only a limited yet growing body of literature examines the health of people like the Bridge Kids and others in IRRs.

In support of this line of reasoning, a small body of research shows there are significant health disparities for people in different *relationship types* (SRR vs. IRR). The findings of these studies show that people in IRRs have elevated levels of psychological distress, greater depressive symptoms, and rate their overall health as poorer than those in SRRs (Barr & Simons, 2014; Bratter & Eschbach, 2006; Tillman & Miller, 2017). One might also expect that by specifically looking at the race of a person's partner as well as the *couple's racial composition* would provide a more nuanced perspective for investigating the health of people in romantic relationships generally, with special emphasis on those in IRRs. Considering the race of each partner reveals that people in some interracial partnerships are at risk of having poorer health than those in same-race relationships but some others seem to benefit from their mixed-race partnership. It has also been discovered these health disparities further vary by the race and gender of the individual and their partner's race (Bratter & Eschbach, 2006; Miller & Kail, 2016; Miller, James, & Roy, 2022; Wong & Penner, 2018). Collectively, this body of litera-ture indicates that a broader understanding for the health of people in roman-tic relationships requires considering the synergistic effects of each partner's sociodemographic characteristics, resources, individual experiences, as well as the dyadic experiences as a couple. However, it still remains unclear as to *why* the well-being of the Bridge Kids and others in IRRs differs from those in SRRs as well as one another. Therefore, it is prudent to examine the possible theoretical explanations for the health disparities between people in SRRs and those in IRRs.

THEORETICAL DETERMINANTS OF THE BRIDGE KIDS' HEALTH

The role race plays in affecting an individual's health, especially racial minorities, cannot be overstated and the impact of race on the health of one's partner is often underestimated. The magnitude of the effect a person's race has on the health of his or her partner is dependent on a number of factors related to their own race and gender, as well as the race of their partner. As one White female married to her Black husband states, "White America needs to stop viewing our black neighbors as second-class citizens. I find that I have experienced some of the discrimination that my husband has tolerated his entire life, although certainly not to the degree he has. It is shameful that race plays such a role in the worth assigned to individuals. It can be very hurtful for me to observe how my husband is treated at times, and it makes me very angry" (Lewis, 2014: p. 23). Accounting for each of these characteristics is especially pertinent for those in IRRs since the bi-directional nature of romantic relationships means the health of an individual and their partner are directly and indirectly effected by each other's racial identity.

The growing prevalence of IRRs, particularly among young adults like the Bridge Kids, means the urgency to investigate and explain their health outcomes is also growing. Currently, there is no proven theoretical explanation for the observed health disparities between people in IRRs and those in SRRs, as researchers have yet to fully explain why people in IRRs tend to have poorer health outcomes than those with same-race partners. It is also unlikely that one theory alone could completely explain such a perplexing topic. With this dilemma in mind, this section focuses on three theories researchers can draw upon to explain the health disparities between people in SRRs and IRRs: 1) the *theory of fundamental causes*; 2) the *social selection hypothesis*, and 3) the *social causation hypothesis*.

The *theory of fundamental causes*, postulates that stratified social positions, such as race and socioeconomic status (SES), contribute to people's unequal exposure to the types of harmful risk factors, social strains, and stressful life events that cause disease, as well as differential access to the resources people use to cope with stress and prevent illness (Link & Phelan, 1995; Phelan, Link, & Tehranifar, 2010; Williams & Collins, 1995; Williams et al., 2019). Racial identity and SES are both considered a fundamental cause of health disparities because race is often a proxy for factors that significantly affect well-being such as a person's socioeconomic status, social environments, stress exposure, and coping resources (LaVeist, 2005; Phelan et al., 2010; Williams et al., 2019). The findings from a robust body of literature support this premise and show there are significant racial disparities in health (Brown & Turner, 2010; Kail & Taylor, 2014; Miller & Taylor, 2012).

The theory of fundamental causes can be used to propose racial disparities in health extend to the well-being of romantically involved people since the health, stressors, and resources of one person in the partnership can affect the overall health of the other. This is particularly applicable to the health of individuals in IRRs who tend to face greater exposure to stressors like discrimination, racism, and microaggressions (Bell & Hastings, 2011; Seshadri & Knudson-Martin, 2013; Solsberry, 1994; Steinbugler, 2012), which in turn increases their risk of having poorer health than those in SRRs. Consequently, the health disparities among romantically involved people are likely to be stratified by differences in the individual's own race, the race of his or her partner, and the couple's racial composition.

The *social selection hypothesis* contends that a person's health influences their choice in romantic partner. That is healthy people are more likely to be in a romantic relationship and maintain their relationship status (Carr &

Springer, 2010; Goldman, 1994). Another way to view this is the healthiest people are seen as the most desirable partners and the unhealthiest are the least desirable partners. With regards to interracial romance, the social selection hypothesis can be used to argue that partner's race may be related to an individual's health because there is a greater likelihood that healthier people from different racial groups form IRRs with one another. As such, healthy people in IRRs are likely to have better health than those in SRRs. Alternatively, it could be argued that the healthiest people select same-race partners, leaving a pool of people with the poorest health from every group who subsequently form IRRs. In this case, unhealthy people are likely to be in IRRs and therefore more likely to have poorer health than those in SRRs.

In contrast, we are not sure if the multitude of factors associated with being in an IRR negatively impacts a person's health. The *social causation hypothesis* contends that romantic partnerships impact health. That is, relationships impact health through the numerous economic, psychological, and social resources and strains associated with the partnership. However, different racial groups have disproportionate access to the financial and psychosocial resources as well as exposure to the stressors and strains that adversely impact their well-being and contribute to racial health disparities (Blendon et al., 2007; Phelan et al., 2010; Turner & Marino, 1994).

In the context of IRRs, the social causation hypothesis suggests that being in an IRR is a risk factor for poor health because some people do not have the resources (economic, psychological, or social) to cope with the social strains and stressors to which people in IRRs are exposed. These effects may vary by the couple's racial composition however, whereby IRRs may benefit the health of minorities with White partners because it provides them with access to the resources and social networks of the dominant White group that they may otherwise not have. In contrast, interracial romance may be more detrimental to the health of Whites who may be forced to deal with racism and racial discrimination, in addition to having a partner who is a racial minority that likely faces such chronic strains and has fewer SES-related coping resources to the partnership. Conversely, IRRs could be detrimental to high SES minorities partnered with low SES Whites and beneficial to Whites when those roles are reversed. This means it is important to look at the stressors to which people in IRRs are exposed as well as the coping resources a person has available to better determine the impact stress exposure and vulnerability to adverse life events have on the health of people in interracial relationships.

Although each of the three theoretical perspectives discussed above can be used to explain health disparities between people in same-race and interracial romantic relationships, there are numerous factors for which these approaches do not account. It is also important to note the lack of longitudinal data with the appropriate measures has made determining social selection or social causation difficult, but two studies using longitudinal data for their analyses (Miller, 2014; Tillman & Miller, 2017), find support for a social causation argument. Given the complexity of assessing the bi-directional and synergistic effects of the interaction between a person's race and gender as well as the race of their partner on the health of individuals in IRRs, it seems especially reasonable to consider that a different approach may be more practical. For these reasons, I believe the Stress Process is a more ideal theoretical framework to examine the association between interracial romance and health.

INTERRACIAL RELATIONSHIP HEALTH MODEL

The sociological study of stress embraces the use of a Stress Process Model (Pearlin, 1989; Pearlin et al., 1981). The stress process theory posits that disparities in health and well-being tend to vary by an individual's social characteristics such as their race, gender, and relationship status (Pearlin, 1989; Pearlin et al., 1981). Variations in social characteristics often translate into differential exposure to stressful life events (e.g., the death of a loved one, job loss, getting married), which in turn can lead to health disparities (Turner, Wheaton, & Lloyd, 1995). Differences in health outcomes may then be explained by mediating factors. For example, experiencing racial discrimination may explain why people in IRRs have lower psychological well-being than those in SRRs. When stressful events arise, people draw upon their available resources to help them cope with unpleasant circumstances. Therefore, accounting for differences in the availability of personal resources (e.g., self-esteem, emotional resilience) and social resources (e.g., emotional support, financial support) someone needs to help them cope with the stressful event and protect their well-being can help explain (mediate) health disparities (Pearlin, 1989; Pearlin et al., 1981). Furthermore, even when people with similar social characteristics are exposed to the same stressors, health outcomes may be moderated (vary) by factors such as race and gender due to the diverse social conditions faced by persons of different races and genders.

Because people in IRRs report experiencing social stressors that those in SRRs do not, suggests the association between relationship type (same-race or interracial) and health may be mediated by differences in social stressors. For these reasons, Miller (2014) used the underlying tenets of the Stress Process (Pearlin, 1981; Turner, 2013) to propose a more nuanced conceptual model for specifically examining health disparities by relationship type and the couple's racial composition. The following sections expand Miller's model to present a more detailed *Interracial Relationship Health Model* (see Figure 3.1). The expanded model includes pathways (indicated by the arrows) conceptualizing the theoretical linkages between relationship type/couple's racial

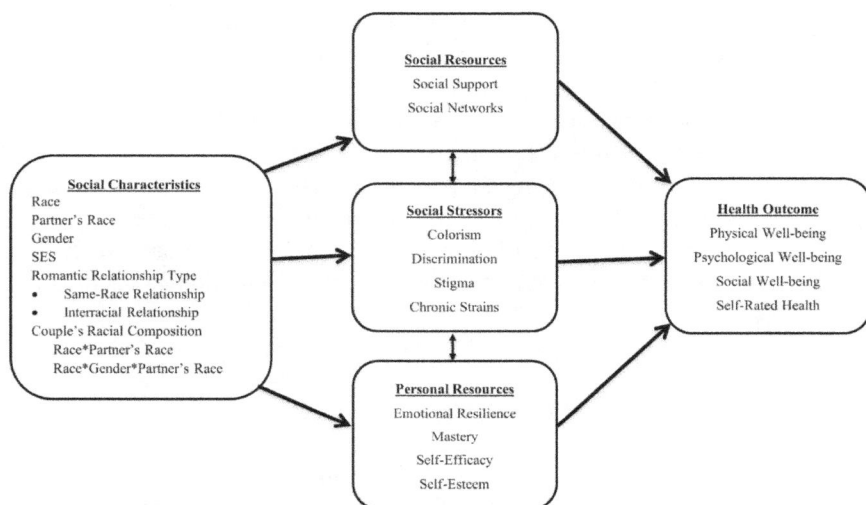

Figure 3.1. Conceptualization of the Interracial Relationship Health Model. Created by the author.

composition and health outcomes that can be mediated and/or moderated by the social stressors to which he or she is exposed, as well as the personal and social coping resources the individual has available. Because it is derived from the stress process framework, this Interracial Relationship Health Model can then be used, and further adapted, to facilitate a more in-depth discussion on the psychosocial mechanisms that affect the well-being of the Bridge Kids and other persons in mixed-race partnerships.

HEALTH OUTCOMES

The World Health Organization (WHO) defines *health* as a person's complete physical, psychological, and social well-being, and not merely the absence of disease or illness (1948). Each dimension of well-being reflects a different aspect of a person's health. Physical well-being, for instance, includes a person's "lifestyle behavior choices to ensure health, avoid preventable diseases and conditions, and to live in a balanced state of body, mind, and spirit" (aana.com, 2022). Psychological well-being refers to some "combination of feeling good and functioning effectively . . . therefore people with high [psychological well-being] report feeling happy, capable, well-supported, satisfied with life, and so on" Winefield et al., 2012: p. 2). The often overlooked social-well-being is "adequate and well-functioning social relationships, adequate social support, little or no social strain, some social participation, social inclusion, in one's society, strong and well-functioning social networks, and perhaps, sexuality as one desires" (Waite, 2018: p. 100).

Although each dimension of health is unique, it is important to keep in mind that they are interdependent, and one aspect of well-being can significantly effect, and be affected by, others. For example, after being diagnosed with cancer (physical well-being), a person may become depressed (psychological well-being), which causes him or her to limit their interactions with family and friends (social well-being). Thus, a holistic approach to understanding health outcomes requires giving a level of attention to each of the three dimensions of health.

SOCIAL WELL-BEING

Social well-being relates to the relationships and circumstances that affect a person's ability to live a healthy life. These conditions include social networks, social integration, social contribution, social coherence, social actualization, and social acceptance (Keyes, 1998; Michaelson, Mahony, & Schifferes, 2012). In terms of their own social well-being, interracially involved young adults perceive having poorer quality relationships with their parents, in which they feel less close and believe their parents care less about them than those in SRRs (Kreager, 2008; Tillman & Miller, 2017; Wang, Kao, & Joyner, 2006). Young adults in IRRs are also less likely to talk to their parents about their romantic relationship or meet the parents of his or her partner (Wang et al. 2006), suggesting they are more likely to hide their relationship because of the perceived lack of acceptance or understanding from their parents. The acceptability of interracial partnerships largely varies by the partner's race (Passel et al., 2010), which is indicative of the social importance of the couple's racial composition (Asian-Black; Native-White; Black-Hispanic; etc.). Furthermore, a lack of social acceptance can signal a lack of trust and comfortability of others as well as elicit a lack of self-acceptance in one's own actions and beliefs (Keyes, 1998), which may deleteriously impact well-being and contribute to health disparities across different racial compositions of interracial couples.

In contrast, people in IRRs typically have family and friends that are interracially involved relatives themselves (Clark-Ibanez & Femlee, 2004; Kao, Joyner, & Balistreri, 2019; Miller et al., 2021) who probably serve as sources of support. This is an important form of social integration because "[h]ealthy individuals feel that they are a part of society. Integration is therefore the extent to which people feel they have something in common with others who constitute their social reality" (Keyes, 1998: p. 122). Similarly, interracially involved persons are likely to have a more racially diverse social network

(Kreager, 2008), that is also supportive of their interracial partnership. As such, there appear to be many factors associated with the social well-being of interracially involved persons that warrant further empirical exploration of this health outcome.

PHYSICAL WELL-BEING

Of the three measures comprising health, the least is known about the physical well-being of interracially involved persons. Beyond the important research on intimate partner violence (Fusco, 2010; Martin et al., 2013), the extant literature has largely overlooked investigating the physical well-being of interracially involved persons. Given the lack of research on addressing this critical health outcome for the interracially involved demographic, I will use a sociological perspective to briefly discuss the impact social stressors may have on the physical well-being of the Bridge Kids and other interracially involved people. To begin, stress is the emotional or physical tension an individual experiences in response to a real or perceived threat (medlineplus. gov, 2021; Smith & Vale, 2006). The source of the stress is called a stressor, which is "the experiential circumstances that give rise to stress" (Pearlin, 1989: p. 243). Social stressors are therefore the social conditions that elicit a stressful response. Moreover, stress is a disturbance to a person's natural state of homeostasis, which in turn triggers the body's allostasis response to resume its homeostatic functioning.

The body's allostasis response is controlled by the hypothalamic-pituitary-adrenal response axis (HPA), which initially involves the detection of a possible threat (stress) by the brain's hypothalamus. This triggers the physiological "fight or flight" response, whereby the pituitary gland releases hormones into the bloodstream as well as "tells" the adrenal gland to release adrenaline and cortisol into the bloodstream, so the person is prepared to deal with the threat by either fighting or running away. After the stressful event subsides, the body needs time to recharge and return to a state of homeostasis, so it is prepared to deal with future stressors. Problems arise, however, when stressful events proliferate, and the body is not given adequate time to recharge between stressors. When the burden on the allostasis system (allostatic load) is too great, the risk of vascular cell inflammation increases, as well as stiffened, scarred, and clogged blood vessels. Such issues are associated with severely adverse physical well-being outcomes including high blood pressure, cardiovascular disease, heart attacks, and strokes (Barr, 2019; Smith & Vale, 2006; Turner, Brown, & Hale, 2017). Thus, social stressors can have significantly harmful effects to a person's physical well-being. Applying the HPA process to people in IRRs, suggests their increased exposure to the unique social stressors related to being in a marginalized romantic relationship puts people in IRRs at greater risk of having poorer physical well-being than those in SRRs, especially if these stressful events frequently occur.

SELF-RATED HEALTH

Self-rated health is a subjective measure of an individual's overall level of mental, physical, and social well-being that World Health Organization (WHO) recommends using as a primary measure for the health and quality of life in the population (Baidin, Gerry, & Kaneva, 2021). Accordingly, self-rated health is a measure that is frequently used to assess a person's overall health status. Since each of the three dimensions of well-being are distinct yet interconnected, it is entirely possible that someone rates their mental health as poor but their overall health as excellent because they view their physical health and social relationships to be in good standing.

Romantic relationships are social in nature and can greatly affect a person's physical and psychological well-being. From this perspective, self-rated health is an important outcome to assess the health of interracially partnered people because the degree to which IRRs are socially accepted is likely to have an impact on the different measures of well-being for each partner. However, only a few studies have examined the self-rated health of people in IRRs and the findings from this limited body of research is inconclusive. On one hand, Barr and Simons (2014) found that interracial couples with one Black and one Nonblack partner (Black-Nonblack pairings) report lower self-rated health than same-race couples. This is an interesting finding because the study examined the health of the interracial couple as a dyad, rather than each partner independently. On the other hand, using nationally representative data pooled from 1997 to 2013, Yu and Zhang (2017) found that White individuals with Black, other-race, and Hispanic spouses, respectively, have 33 percent, 23 percent, and 8 percent lower odds of reporting better self-rated health than those with White spouses. Another study using nationally representative census data not only found that White persons with White spouses reported having the highest self-rated health, but racial minorities with same-race spouses were also between 14 percent (Blacks) and 27 percent (Asians and Hispanics) less likely to report their self-rated health is better than their same-race counterparts with White spouses (Miller & Kail, 2016). Along similar lines, Miller, James, and Roy (2022) found that Black, Hispanic, and White men all reported having the highest self-rated health when partnered with a Black woman. These findings suggest that, depending on the specific race and gender of the couple's composition, interracial romance is actually better for the overall health of some people. Still, the lack of research and disparate results point to the need for much more research addressing the self-rated health of those in IRRs.

SOCIAL CHARACTERISTICS

Examining the association between social characteristics and health allows researchers to more fully investigate the social determinants that affect the health of the Bridge Kids and others in IRRs. A limited, but growing, body of research demonstrates an individual's *relationship type* (SRR vs. IRR) is a significant predictor of health, as people in IRRs generally have an elevated risk of being diagnosed with anxiety, depression, and psychological distress than those in SRRs (Barr & Simons, 2014; Bratter & Eschbach, 2006; Miller, 2014; Tillman & Miller, 2017; Miller, James, and Roy, 2022). The evidence for self-rated is much more mixed and shows that, dependent on the couple's racial composition, interracial romance is beneficial to the self-rated health of some and harmful to the health of others (Barr & Simons, 2014; Miller et al., 2022; Miller & Kail, 2016). In sum, the extant literature clearly indicates that, by virtue of having a partner with a different racial background, people in IRRs generally face a greater risk of mental illness and other questionable health outcomes.

Still, there is no ubiquitous application of these findings to everyone in IRRs as there are significant health disparities by a person's race and gender as well as the race of their partner. For example, Bratter and Eschbach (2006) found that intermarried people with a Black or Native American spouse respectively have 70 percent and 114 percent greater likelihood of being psychologically distressed than their same-race counterparts in same-race marriages. Wong and Penner (2018) found that, in terms of the initial health effects of a single person entering a romantic relationship (partner selection), single men and women that enter a SRR receive the psychological benefits generally associated with being in a romantic partnership but those who enter IRRs do not.

Understanding these health outcomes become even more complex when using an intersectionality approach that assesses the combined effects of multiple social characteristics such as: (1) the individual's race and gender (race*gender); (2) the individual's race and their partner's race (race*partner race); (3) the individual's gender and their partner's race (gender*partner race); and (4) the individual's race and gender as well as their partner's race (race*gender*partner race). There are fewer consistencies in the findings of, and fewer studies that have examined, the health of persons in IRRs when accounting for these multiple characteristics. Some findings show that forming an IRR is worse for the psychological well-being of Black men and Hispanic women (Wong & Penner, 2018), and interracial marriage is more detrimental to the psychological well-being of White women, Hispanic women, and Hispanic men than those in same-race marriages (Bratter & Eschbach 2006). Also, persons that are interracially involved with Black or Native American partners face an increased risk of having poorer psychological well-being, especially White women and White men (Bratter & Eschbach, 2006; Wong & Penner, 2018).

Other studies find that IRRs are beneficial to the psychological well-being of Hispanic men (Wong & Penner, 2018) as well as the self-rated health of Hispanic men and women who have Black partners (Miller et al., 2022). There is also evidence suggesting minorities in interracial relationships with White partners generally have better self-rated health than those in SRRs (Miller & Kail, 2016). When accounting for the individual's race and gender as well as their partner's race, Miller and colleagues (2022) discover that women (White, Black, and Hispanic) partnered with Hispanic men have the greatest risk of being depressed, and men (White, Black, and Hispanic) partnered with Black women have the highest self-rated health. It is therefore clear that the race and gender of an individual and their partner (*couple's racial composition*) have a profound impact on the health of the individual *and* their partner. Yet, we still do not fully understand *why* the race of one's partner is linked to an individual's health or the extent to which well-being varies by the couple's racial composition.

SES differences may at least partially explain the disparities in the risks and benefits of interracial romance generally, and across specific couple's racial composition specifically. Low SES is generally associated with a lack of health insurance, lack of healthcare and healthcare resources, shorter life expectancy, and worse overall health (Barr, 2019; LaVeist, 2005). The correlation between SES and an individual's health extends to romantic relationships as well since married people with the lowest SES tend to have poorer health than those in the higher categories (Karney, 2021; Wilson, 2001). Among married couples, household income varies by the couple's racial composition whereby people in interracial relationships are usually more educated and have higher incomes than those in same-race relationships (Wang, 2012). Such differences suggest the association between couple's racial composition and health likely varies by SES as well, which means differences in SES could help explain the health disparities between people in SRRs and IRRs.

Racial minorities with White partners are generally more educated and have higher income than those in SRRs (Wang, 2012), implies minorities in IRRs with White partners may gain a *partner premium* resulting in better health than those in SRRs. Alternatively, it is possible that White individuals in lower SES households with minority partners receive a *partner penalty* that makes them more vulnerable to poor health outcomes. This view is supported by Bratter and Eschbach (2006) who found that about half of the greater psychological distress reported by intermarried White women was explained by their disadvantaged socioeconomic position relative to White women in same-race marriages. Given the consistently strong association between SES and health contrasted by the significant lack of research investigating the effects of SES on the observed racial disparities by couple's racial composition, suggests the lack of knowledge on this topic is an area that deserves being addressed by future research.

SOCIAL STRESSORS

Accounting for the impact of social stressors on people's lives is essential for comprehending the health of the Bridge Kids and others in IRRs. *Social stressors* are those circumstances or interactions that lead to occasional (acute) or frequent (chronic) feelings of stress (Pearlin 1989). Being in an IRR is a marginalized status that often leads to the stigmatization of interracial couples, thereby exposing individuals in interracial relationships to a unique set of social stressors not experienced by those in SRRs. Many individuals that cross racial lines for romance report being exposed to racism, discrimination, and stigmatization from those that disapprove of amalgamated partnerships (Bell & Hastings, 2015; Bonilla-Silva & Forman, 2000; Childs, 2005; Yancey, 2007). It is therefore important to assess the impact exposure to social stressors has on the health of people in interracial relationships.

CHRONIC STRAINS

The general lack of acceptance for interracial romance can lead to other types of stressors experienced by people in IRRs. *Chronic strains* involve "the relatively enduring problems, conflicts, and threats that many people face in their daily lives" (Pearlin, 1989: p. 245). The strain for interracial couples is generally associated with the disapproval of interracial romance by society, family, and friends that creates tension and conflict for interracially involved persons (Lawton, Foeman, & Braz, 2012). Disapproval of a one's IRR by their family and friends can lead to strained interactions and even the loss of those relationships. Strain from family, friends, or society could also put undue stress on an interracial partnership to the point of causing the couple to break up. As one young adult stated, their IRR ended "because the 'outside' disapproved, especially my family which put a lot of strain on the relationship" (Femlee, 2001: p. 1279). This can be especially detrimental to one's health because a romantic breakup is associated with an increase of depressive symptoms among young adults (Miller 2014; Simon & Barrett 2010), and the instability of marital divorce is linked to poor mental health and lower life satisfaction among adults (Symoens, Colman, & Bracke, 2014).

In addition, the general lack of social acceptance from the relatively large proportion of the U.S. population that disapprove of interracial romance (Carroll, 2007; Passel et al., 2010), is yet another social stressor faced by individuals in IRRs. The widespread lack of acceptance for interracial romance means that, as stated by a Hispanic male married to a White female, interracial couples should be "prepared to accept prejudice from those you would least suspect it from" (Lewis, 2014: p. 22). Thus, the general lack of acceptance is likely to contribute to people in IRRs being exposed to unique social stressors that can negatively impact their health in a multitude of ways and contribute to the health disparities between those in SRRs and those in IRRs.

STIGMA

Erving Goffman referred to stigmatized people as those individuals who are not fully accepted by society (Goffman 1963, Link & Phelan 2001), and interracially involved people recognize their relationships are more marginalized than "traditional" same-race partnerships (Lehmiller & Agnew, 2006). Like racism and discrimination, *social stigma* is a stressor that can negatively affect a person's social and psychological well-being (Hatzenbuehler et al., 2013), which may in turn manifest as poorer health outcomes for socially stigmatized persons (Bostwick et al., 2014). The subsequent stigma individuals in IRRs perceive from family, friends, and society is associated with them perceiving elevated levels of discrimination (Rosenthal & Starks, 2015), which is another social stressor that is harmful to one's health.

DISCRIMINATION

Racial *discrimination* is as the differential treatment of members of minority groups through both institutional arrangements and interpersonal social interactions (Williams & Williams-Morris, 2000). Exposure to racism and discrimination is also associated with greater depressive symptomatology (Brown et al., 2000; Miller et al., 2013; Williams et al., 2019). The effects of being mistreated because of their relationship type may be worse for interracially involved Whites, who are protected by white privilege and therefore otherwise less likely to experience racial discrimination. In contrast, because of their race, minorities are often socialized on how to endure a lifetime of discrimination (Hughes et al., 2017; Tran & Lee, 2010). Examining the effects of racial discrimination is especially relevant to people in IRRs considering one or both partners may be discriminated against for being a racial minority, or the couple is mistreated by those who oppose such relationships. For instance, both partners in Black-White marriages often report perceiving being treated differently than couples with other racial compositions, further revealing the significant influence race continues to have in contemporary U.S. society (Lewis, 2014). Accordingly, the health of interracially partnered Whites could be more negatively affected by discrimination than their minority partner.

COLORISM

Race further impacts the health of interracially involved people in terms of colorism. *Colorism* refers to allocating social privilege or prejudice based on skin tone, whereby lighter skinned individuals are viewed more favorably than darker skinned persons (Burton et al., 2010). Since people with darker skin tend to be viewed more negatively by members of our society, it's not surprising that people in IRRs with Black partners perceive their social interactions as more negative than those with lighter skinned partners (Lewis, 2014). Accordingly, people interracially involved with a Black partner generally have poorer psychological well-being (Bratter & Eschbach, 2006; Kroeger & Williams, 2011). Thus, the prejudicial treatment associated with colorism is another significant stressor that may affect the health of interracially involved persons.

Since colorism is considered a form of prejudice or discrimination based on an individual's skin tone whereby darker skinned people are treated less favorably than those with lighter complexions, people with different skin complexions are differentially impacted by its effects (Hannon, 2015; NCCJ, 2021). Particularly, darker skinned people not only perceive being discriminated against more often (Monk, 2015) but, among both Blacks and Black-Hispanics specifically, those with darker skin tones also have worse mental health (see Cuevas, Dawson, & Williams, 2016) and lower self-esteem (Thompson & Keith, 2001) than those with lighter complexions. Other research links darker skin tones to higher allostatic load (Cobb et al., 2016), hypertension and other mental and physical health disparities (see Monk, 2021). This suggests that interracial couples where at least one of the partners has darker skin are more likely to deal with adverse health issues due to their exposure to stressors associated with colorism.

PERSONAL RESOURCES

Emotional Resilience

Everyone goes through some form of stress and adversity in life, but the affects differ as people endure and adapt to stressful circumstances and events in different ways. *Emotional resilience* is a form of positive psychological capital that is characterized as having the ability to adjust to the changing demands of stressful experiences (APA, 2012; Lloyd, Katz, & Pronk, 2016). For example, emotional resilience includes adapting to work and financial stressors, chronic strains, tragedy, health problems, family, and relationship problems (APA, 2012). Since some stressful events are unavoidable, like the death of a loved one or becoming seriously ill, a person's ability to bounce back after facing such hardships without emotionally breaking down is equally as important as their ability to cope with stress and trauma. The inability to bounce back can have deleterious effects on one's well-being, as resilience helps mitigate the social, psychological, and physical health consequences of disadvantage across the life course (Crosnoe & Elder, 2004; Krause, 2020). A person's aptitude of being emotionally resilient to stress and stressors can also be developed over time as individuals adjust to experiences of stress exposure or employ emotional resilience building strategies (Davis, 2009; Lloyd et al., 2016). Thus, emotional resilience gives a person a level of control over how they handle the stress and stressors that subsequently impacts their health and well-being.

Emotional resilience is especially important to individuals in IRRs because there are significant racial differences in emotional resilience such that minorities, particularly Blacks, have greater emotional resilience than Whites (Bartley et al., 2019; Youssef et al., 2016). Furthermore, people in stressful and psychologically distressing professions such as nurses and social workers who have high emotional resilience and frequently exposed to stressful circumstances are able to cope with their own stress as well as help others do the same without harming their own psychological well-being (Grant & Kinman, 2013). This suggests that, in the context of a romantic relationship, if one partner has high emotional resilience, he or she can probably help their partner cope with stressful events while maintaining their own positive psychological well-being. For those in IRRs, the high emotional resilience of racial minorities, particularly Blacks, can help themselves and their partner, better cope with the stressors associated with interracial romance. Over time, the person with higher resilience can help their partner strengthen his or her resiliency to race-based stressors so the well-being of both people is better protected.

Mastery

There tend to be some aspects of life over which most people want some, if not total, control. For example, students might study with the belief that doing so will earn them good grades, or employees may work extra hard because they believe it will earn them a raise in pay or status. However, despite their greatest efforts, people are sometimes unable to control their social environments or the things that happen in their lives. Sometimes students that study get poor grades and hard workers are not guaranteed a pay raise or promotion. Still, the belief that one can control the circumstances influencing their life chances is referred to as *mastery* (Pearlin & Schooler, 1978). Mastery is a coping resource that is positively correlated to health outcomes whereby people who believe they have a greater sense of control, or mastery, over the circumstances in their lives report having better psychological well-being than those with less control (Assari, 2019; Miller et al., 2013). Mastery is also important for people with chronic physical illnesses like cardiovascular and kidney disease because it promotes improved coping and health outcomes (Schipper & Abma, 2011; Surtees et al., 2010). Those with higher mastery have better health because they tend to view themselves as being competent people who possess the skills that can help them cope with, and resolve, difficult issues.

Having a sense of control over the circumstances of one's life is a particularly salient coping resource for people that are interracially involved. For one, women perceive having less mastery than men (Tyndall & Christie-Mizell, 2016; Zalta & Chambless, 2012), which suggests women are less able than men to cope with the circumstances they cannot control. The lessened ability to cope with being exposed to the additional stressors associated with interracial romance over which they lack control such as disapproval from their family (Bell & Hastings, 2015; Miller et al., 2021) or being discriminated against in public (cbsnews.com, 2017), may make interracially involved women more vulnerable to poor health outcomes than men and women that are in SRRs. Similarly, the health of members of socially disadvantaged groups with less power, like racial minorities, may also be more vulnerable to the distinct stressors related to interracial romance if they believe they lack the ability to control their experiences and have fewer resources to avoid or resolve problems like being unfairly treated at a restaurant or by law enforcement officers. Conversely, interracially partnered individuals with a high level of mastery may purposively choose to reside in more racially integrated neighborhoods or befriend other interracial couples (Villazor, 2018), which in turn could protect their well-being.

There is also a robust association between mastery and SES such that those with higher SES also perceive having greater mastery over their life circumstances (Miller et al., 2013; Tyndall & Christie-Mizell 2016). The clear disparities in SES by couple's racial composition (Wang, 2012) suggests at the dyadic level, there may be significant differences in mastery by the couple's racial compositions, which in turn may contribute to health disparities at both the individual and dyadic levels. This may be particularly relevant to Blacks and Hispanics with White partners as those couples tend to have higher SES than their Black and Hispanic counterparts in SRRs. The greater sense of mastery possessed by men and persons in higher SES households could allow those individuals to feel they are more in control of their life circumstances and life chances, which in turn protects their well-being, especially interracially partnered men as well as Blacks and Hispanics with White partners.

Self-Efficacy

Social learning theory presupposes fear of potential stressors elicits a cognitive and physiological response that increases a person's vulnerability to the adverse effects of stress. Through their experiences of coping with those situations, however, people learn to perceive them as less threatening, become less frightened, and thus become less vulnerable to the harmful effects of the stressor (Bandura, 1977). Therefore, developing effective strategies and behaviors to handle stressful situations is an important coping skill. Such a coping ability reflects a person's *self-efficacy*, which is the expectation or belief that one's behavior or particular course of action will lead to their desired outcome (Bandura, 1977). People with stronger perceived self-efficacy are also willing to cope with adverse circumstances longer and reinforce their efficacy by confronting and eliminating their fears, whereas those that are unable to fully cope remain fearful of such situations. Given that people with high self-efficacy are less fearful and more willing to endure stressful situations longer than those with less efficacy, it is not surprising that self-efficacy is positively related to both physical and psychological well-being (Riggio et al., 2013; Tsay & Chao, 2002; Weisskirch, 2017). Thus, people that develop high self-efficacy by learning to cope with their fears have better physical health like lower heart failure rates and better mental health in terms of fewer symptoms of anxiety and depression than those with less self-efficacy.

The development of self-efficacy as a coping resource is especially important for romantically involved individuals since it positively related to relationship satisfaction and expectations of relationship success and related to more adept partners engaging in relationship promoting behaviors (Riggio et al., 2013; Weiser & Weigel, 2016). This implies the level of a person's self-efficacy influences how they treat their romantic partner, as well as the level of strain and relationship satisfaction each partner perceives. Self-efficacy also influences one's choices of activities and environments whereby "[p]eople fear and tend to avoid threatening situations they believe exceed their coping skills, whereas they get involved in activities and behave assuredly when they judge themselves capable of handling situations that would otherwise be intimidating" (Bandura, 1977: p. 194). In other words, people try not put themselves in situations they believe will be too stressful for them to handle. This suggests that if one or both partners in an IRR has low self-efficacy, perhaps he or she may intentionally avoid stressful situations like family gatherings with people they know oppose of their relationship, but those with high self-efficacy might not view such situations as threatening to themselves or their relationship. Learning how to acquire such a coping mechanism can be beneficial to the health of people in IRRs because according to the vicarious experience of self-efficacy, "[s]eeing others perform threatening activities without adverse consequences can generate expectations in observers that they too will improve if they intensify and persist in their efforts" (Bandura, 1977: p. 197). Consequently, even if only one partner has high self-efficacy at the onset of the relationship, the other partner can learn to develop this valuable coping skill as well.

Self-Esteem

How a person views and feels about themselves is another essential personal resource for protecting one's health against the negative effects of stress. *Self-esteem* describes a person's perceived negative or positive feelings of their own self-worth, value, self-confidence, self-appreciation, and self-identity (Mann et al., 2004). "Positive self-esteem is not only seen as a basic feature of mental health, but also as a protective factor that contributes to better health and positive social behavior through its role as a buffer against the impact of negative influences. It is seen to actively promote healthy functioning as reflected in life aspects such as achievements, success, satisfaction, and the ability to cope with diseases like cancer and heart disease" (Mann et al., 2004: pp. 357–58). A review of the existing literature shows people with higher self-esteem generally engage in healthier behaviors like less substance use, fewer sexual partners, eating a more nutritious diet, and being more physically active (Arsandaux et al., 2020). Thus, positive self-esteem is a significant coping resource that is associated with better health and health behaviors (Mann et al., 2004; Marmot, 2003).

Having a positive evaluation of oneself and self-identity is especially important for the health of individuals in IRRs. High self-esteem is beneficial in romantic relationships as it is positively associated with relationship satisfaction (Erol & Orth, 2017). There are racial differences in self-esteem, however, with Blacks having higher self-esteem than Whites, Hispanics, and Asians (Sprecher, Brooks, & Avogo, 2013; Tobin et al., 2021), which may contribute to health disparities between Blacks and their partners in IRRs. There are also significant gender differences whereby men typically have higher self-esteem than women (Sprecher et al., 2013). Among adults with low self-esteem, both men and women feel more loved and accepted by their partner when their professional career is successful, but women feel less love and acceptance when they experienced a professional failure (Murray et al., 2006). That is, the health of women with low self-esteem is especially vulnerable to the adverse effects of social stressors. As such, having high self-esteem may be an exceedingly significant personal resource for interracially involved persons, who face more stressors than those in SRRs, especially Nonblacks and women.

SOCIAL RESOURCES

Social Support

When stressful events arise, people draw on their different available coping resources to help them deal with the psychological distress that rises from the situation. One resource that is of profound importance to protecting the vulnerability of people's health from the deleterious effects of stress and stressors is social support. *Social support* is the perception that a person is loved, valued, and esteemed by others, as well as the interpersonal social resources he or she can draw upon to help them cope with stressful events and circumstances (Thoits, 2011; Turner & Turner, 1999). There are multiple types of support a person can receive from their social relationships including *emotional support* (i.e., love, trust, and empathy), *instrumental support* (i.e., financial assistance and tangible services), *informational support* (i.e., advice and problem solving), and *appraisal support* (i.e., constructive feedback for self-evaluation and decision making) (Heaney & Israel, 2008; House, 1987). Regardless of which type, provisions of social support are always intended to be helpful and beneficial. Accordingly, social support is positively related to health and well-being (Heany & Israel, 2008; Ozbay et al., 2007; Thoits, 2011). Social support from family and friends is particularly important as studies show that, compared to those who score low on this coping mechanism, people who perceive high levels of support from family and friends report fewer symptoms of depression and anxiety (Miller & Taylor, 2012; Thoits, 2011; Thomas, Liu, & Umberson, 2017). Therefore, when stressful events occur, people are likely to perceive their family and friends will give them the social support they need to successfully cope with the distressing circumstances.

Social support is an especially essential coping resource for romantically involved persons. Thoits (1995) considers romantic partners a confidant and one of the most important sources of social support. Since Thoits does not make the distinction that the support of a partner only benefits people in SRRs, I presume that the health benefits of partner support extend to those in IRRs as well. The health benefits of social support may differ by the couple's racial composition, however, for several reasons. For one, Blacks perceive having more support than Whites (Tobin et al., 2021), which likely helps protect the well-being of interracially involved Blacks from the social stressors associated with mixed-race relationships. Another reason is that when stressful events arise, men rely more on their partners for support (Waite & Gallagher, 2000), whereas women seek emotional support from their partner as well as their family and friends (Day & Livingston, 2003; Dykstra & Fokkema, 2007). Given that people who perceive their family to be more supportive have better mental and physical well-being than those that believe their family is less supportive (Shim et al., 2012; Tillman & Miller, 2017), suggests perceived social support from family and friends is more protective of a woman's health regardless of her partner's race. Furthermore, shifts in popular culture that have made seeing interracial couples in movies, television shows, and commercials become normative, may be perceived as a form of appraisal support that helps interracially involved individuals view their relationships as socially acceptable rather than stigmatized. Leaning on their romantic partner, family, and friends as well as perceiving their relationship to be less stigmatized and more socially accepted, may therefore help reduce the stress and protect the well-being of people in IRRs.

Social Networks

Humans are social creatures whose lives and well-being are deeply affected by their interpersonal social connections. *Social networks* refer to the "linkages between people that may or may not provide social support and that may serve functions other than providing support" (Heaney & Israel, 2008: p. 190). Social networks are therefore distinct from social support in that their context is much broader and can involve negative consequences such as interrelationship conflict, role strain, misunderstandings, or poor advice that can increase stress and contribute to poor health outcomes (Wright, 2016). A person's social networks can affect health through a variety of mechanisms including the provision of *social support* (both perceived and actual), *social influence* (e.g., norms, social control, conformity), *social interactions*, *person-to-person contacts* (e.g., pathogen exposure, violence), *access to resources* (e.g., money, jobs, information), and *influencing behavioral risks* (e.g., smoking, drug abuse, exercising) (Heaney & Israel, 2008; Smith & Christakis, 2008). Thus, social networks may affect the occurrence of, and recovery from, disease and illness through its influences on preventative health behaviors, illness behaviors, and sick-role behaviors (Heaney & Israel, 2008).

As the prevalence of interracial romance continues to increase, the likelihood of a people having one or more interracially involved persons in their social network also increases. People's social networks are therefore becoming increasingly important for those in IRRs. Heaney and Israel (2008) propose three advantages of using a social network approach to examine health which are distinct from the social support approach that I believe aptly extends to the study of IRRs. First, the social network approach can *incorporate characteristics of various social relationships* beyond just the support they provide. Specific to the Bridge Kids and others in IRRs, this means a social network approach can investigate, for example, how their health is affected by factors such as the racial composition of the couple, their parents' friendship networks, or the prevalence of interracial romance within their family. Second, a social network approach *allows for understanding how changes in one social relationship affects others*. This could entail, for example, examining whether a childbirth impacts the relationship Bridge Kids have with their family members, or if more members of the person's network subsequently become interracially involved themselves. Third, a social network approach can *account for the influence network characteristics have on the quality and quantity of social support they provide*. For example, do the Bridge Kids lose support or close connections across their entire social network, or specific types of support such as financial assistance (instrumental support) or relationship advice from family and friends (informational support), when they become interracially involved, which in turn may increase their vulnerability to the stress associated with their IRR. Additionally, close-knit and homogeneous networks not only provide emotional and instrumental support, but also exert more influence on members to conform to network norms (Heany & Israel, 2008). This suggests people risk losing social support from their social network if they do not conform to the network's expectations. It therefore stands to reason that, as the prevalence of interracial romance increases, understanding the health of interracially involved persons can be greatly advanced by examining the effects social networks have on their health.

CONCLUSION

In sum, the vast majority of people want to live a long, healthy life and, as the prevalence of interracial romance continues to increase, examining the well-being and factors that affect the health of those in interracial relationships is becoming a much more prominent social issue. The relatively limited body of research investigating this topic suggests people in IRRs generally have worse well-being than those in same-race relationships, but these differences vary by the health outcome of interest as well as the couple's racial composition. In fact, some research finds that people in IRRs have better health than those in SRRs, which suggests the racial disparities in health among those in romantic relationships, which is the majority of the adult population, may be related to the race of a person's partner. To properly address this issue, much more research needs to be conducted that examines the health of the Bridge Kids and others in IRRs.

It is also worth noting that well-being during adolescence and young adulthood is strongly associated with their well-being in later adulthood (Lewinsohn et al., 2003). This is not going away since interracial romance continues to become more common and is most prevalent among the youngest adults. Drawing attention to these issues now can help provide researchers, teachers, and health practitioners with a unique lens for examining current health trends and predicting future health outcomes in our society. Extending this area of research will also allow for the implementation of strategies that will help the Bridge Kids live longer and happier lives.

REFERENCES

American Association of Nurse Anesthesiology. (2022). *Physical Well-Being.* https://www.aana.com/practice/health-and-wellness-peer-assistance/about-health-wellness/physical-well-being.

American Psychological Association. (2012). *Building your resilience.* https://www.apa.org/topics/resilience.

Arsandaux, J., Montagni, I., Macalli, M., Bouteloup, V., Tzourio, C., & Galera, C. (2020). Health Risk Behaviors and Self-Esteem Among College Students: Systematic Review of Quantitative Studies. International *Journal of Behavioural Medicine, 27*, 142–59.

Assari, S. (2019). High sense of mastery reduces psychological distress for African American women but not African American men. *Archives of General Internal Medicine, 3*(1), 5–9.

Baidin, V., Gerry, C. J., & Kaneva, M. (2021). How Self-Rated is Self-Rated Health? Exploring the Role of Individual and Institutional Factors in Reporting

Heterogeneity in Russia,*Social Indicators Research: An International and Interdisciplinary Journal for Qualityof-Life Measurement, 155*(2), 675–96.

Bandura, A. (1977). Self-efficacy: Toward a Unifying Theory of Behavioral Change. *Psychological Review, 84*(2), 191–215.

Barr, A. B., & Simons. R. L. (2014). A Dyadic Analysis of Relationships and Health: Does Couple-Level Context Condition Partner Effects?. *Journal of Family Psychology, 28(*4): 448–59.

Barr, D. A. (2019). *Health Disparities in the United States: Social class, race, ethnicity, and the social determinants of health.* Johns Hopkins University Press.

Bartley, E. J., Hossain, N, I., Gravlee, C. C., Sibille, K. T., Terry, E. L., Vaughn, I. A., Cardoso, J. S., Booker, S. Q., Glover, T. L., Goodin, B. R., Sotolongo, A., Thompson, K. A., Bulls, H. W., Staud, R., Edberg, J. C., Bradley, L. A., & Filingim, R. B. (2019). Race/Ethnicity Moderates the Association Between Psychosocial Resilience and Movement-Evoked Pain in Knee Osteoarthritis. *ACR Open Rheumatology, 1*(1), 16–25.

Bell, G. C., & Hastings, S. O. (2015). Exploring Parental Approval and Disapproval for Black and White Interracial Couples. *Journal of Social Issues, 71*(4), 755–71.

Blendon, R. J., Buhr, T., Cassidy, E. F., Perez, D. J., Hunt, K. A., Fleischfresser, Benson, J. M., & Hermann, M.J. (2007). Disparities in Health: Perspectives of a Multi-Ethnic, *Multi-Racial America. Health Affairs, 26*(5), 1437–47.

Bonilla-Silva, E., & Forman, T. A. (2000). 'I Am Not a Racist But . . . ': Mapping White College Students' Racial Ideology in the USA. *Discourse & Society, 11*(1), 50–85.

Bostwick, W. B., Boyd, C. J., Hughes, T. L., & West, B. (2014). Discrimination and Mental Health Among Lesbian, Gay, and Bisexual Adults in the United States. *American Journal of Orthopsychiatry 84*(1): 35–45.

Bratter, J., & Eschbach, K. (2006). What about the couple? Interracial marriage and psychological distress. *Social Science Research, 35*, 1025–47.

Brown, R. L., & Turner, R. J. (2010). Physical Disability and Depression: Clarifying Racial/Ethnic Contrasts. *Journal of Aging and Health, 22*(7), 977–1000.

Brown, T. N., Williams, D. R., Jackson, J. S., Neighbors, H. W., Torres, M., Sellers, S. L., & Brown, K. T. (2000). Being Black and Feeling Blue: the mental health consequences of racial discrimination. *Race and Society, 2*(2), 117–31.

Burton, L. M, Bonilla-Silva, E., Victor, R. Rose, B., & Freeman, E. H. (2010). Critical Race Theories, Colorism, and the Decade's Research on Families of Color. *Journal of Marriage and Family, 72*(3), 440–59.

Carr, D., & Springer, K. W. (2010). Advances in Families and Health Research in the 21st Century. *Journal of Marriage and Family, 72*(3), 743–61.

Carroll, J. (2007, August 16). Most Americans Approve of Interracial Marriage. *Gallup.* http://www.gallup.com/poll/28417/Most-Americans-Approve-Interracial-Marriages.aspx.

CBSNews.com. (2017, June 12). *50 years later, interracial couples still face hostility from strangers.* https://www.cbsnews.com/news/50-years-loving-case-interracial-couples-still-face-hostility-from-strangers/.

Centers for Medicare and Medicaid Services. https://www.cms.gov/Research-Statistics -Data-and-Systems/Statistics-Trends-and-Reports/NationalHealthExpendData/Nat ionalHealthAccountsHistorical.

Childs, E. C. (2005). Looking Behind the Stereotypes of the Angry Black Woman: An Exploration of Black Women's Responses to Interracial Relationships. *Gender & Society, 19*(4), 544–61.

Clark-Ibanez, M., & Felmlee, D. (2004). Interethnic Relationships: The Role of Social Network Diversity. *Journal of Marriage and Family, 66*(2):293–305.

Clavél, F.D., Cutrona, C.E., & Russell, D.W. (2017). United and Divided by Stress: How Stressors Differentially Influence Social Support in African American Couples Over Time. *Personality and Social Psychology Bulletin, 43*(7), 1050–64.

Cobb, R. J., Thomas, C. S., Pirtle, W. N. L., & Darity Jr. W. A. (2016). Self-Identified Race, Socially Assigned Skin Tone, and Adult Physiological Dysregulation: Assessing Multiple Dimensions of 'Race' in Health Disparities Research, *SSM-Population Health, 2,* 595–602.

Crosnoe, R., & Elder, G. H., Jr. (2004). Family dynamics, supportive relationships, and educational resilience during adolescence. Journal of Family Issues, 25(5), 571–602.

Cuevas, A. G., Dawson, B. A., & Williams, D. R. (2016). Race and Skin Color in Latino Health: An Analytic Review. *American Journal of Public Health, 106*(12), 2131–36.

Davis, M. C. (2009). Building emotional resilience to promote health. *American Journal of Lifestyle Medicine, 3*(1 suppl), 60S–63S.

Day, A. L., & Livingstone, H. A. (2003). Gender differences in perceptions of stress-ors and utilization of social support among university students. *Canadian Journal of Behavioural Science, 35*(2), 73–83.

Dystra, P.A., & Fokkema, T. (2007). Social and Emotional Loneliness Among Divorced and Married Men and Women: Comparing the Deficit and Cognitive Perspectives. *Basic and Applied Social Psychology, 29*(1), 1–12.

Erol, R. Y., & Orth, U. (2017). Self-esteem and the quality of romantic relationships *European Psychologist, 21*(4), 274–83.

Femlee, D. H. (2001). No Couple is an Island: A Social Network Perspective on Dyadic Stability. *Social Forces, 79*(4), 1259–87.

Fusco R. A. (2010). Intimate partner violence in interracial couples: a comparison to white and ethnic minority monoracial couples. *Journal of Interpersonal Violence, 25*(10), 1785–800.

Goffman, Erving. (1963). *Stigma.* New York: Simon & Schuster.

Goldman, N. (1994). Social Inequalities in Health: Disentangling the Underlying Mechanisms. *Annals of New York Academy of Sciences, 954*(1), 118–39.

Grant, L., & Kinman, G. (2013). Emotional Resilience in the Helping Professions and How It Can Be Enhanced. *Health and Social Care Education, 3*(1), 23–34. DOI:10.11120/hsce.2014.00040.

Hannon, L. (2015). White Colorism. *Social Currents 2*(1): 12–21.

Hatzenbuehler, M. L., Phelan, J. C., & Link, B. G. (2013). Stigma as a Fundamental Cause of Population Health Inequalities. *American Journal of Public Health, 103*, 813–21.

Heaney, C. A., & Israel, B. A. (2008). Social networks and social support. In K. Glanz, B. K. Rimer, & K. Viswanath (Eds.), Health behavior and health education: Theory, research, and practice (pp. 189–210). Jossey-Bass.

Herman, M. R., & Campbell, M. E. (2012). I wouldn't, but you can: Attitudes toward interracial relationships. *Social Science Research, 41*, 343–58.

House, J. S. (1987). Social support and social structure. *Sociological Forum, 2*(1), 135–46.

Hughes, D., Harding, J., Niwa, E. Y., & Toro, J. D. (2017). Racial Socialization and Racial Discrimination as Intra-and Intergroup Processes. In book: *The Wiley Handbook of Group Processes in Children and Adolescents* (pp. 241–68).

Human Genome Project. (2019). The Human Genome Project. *National Human Genome Research Institute.* https://www.genome.gov/human-genome-project.

Jia, H., & Lubetkin, E. I. (2020). Life expectancy and active life expectancy by marital status among older U.S. adults: Results from the U.S. Medicare Health Outcome Survey (HOS). *SSM-Population Health, 12*, 1–9.

Jones, J. M. (2005). Most Americans Approve of Interracial Dating. *Gallup.* Available at: http://www.gallup.com/poll/19033/Most-Americans-Approve-Interracial-Dating.aspx.

Kail, B. L., & Taylor, M. G. (2014). Cumulative Inequality and Racial Disparities in Health: Private Insurance Coverage and Black/White Differences in Functional Limitations, The Journals of Gerontology: Series B, 69(5), 798–808.

Kansky, J. (2018). What's love got to do with it?: Romantic relationships and well-being. In E. Diener, S. Oishi, & L. Tay (Eds.), *Handbook of well-being.* DEF Publishers.

Kao, G., Joyner, K., & Balistreri, K. S. (2019). *The Company We Keep: Interracial Friendships from Adolescence to Adulthood.* Russell Sage Foundation.

Karney, Benjamin R. 2021. Socioeconomic Status and Intimate Relationships. *Annual Review of Psychology, 72*: 2.1–2.24.

Keyes, C. L. M. (1998). Social Well-Being. *Social Psychology Quarterly, 61*(2), 121–40.

Khodarahimi, S. (2015). The Role of Marital Status in Emotional Intelligence, Happiness,

Optimism and Hope. *Intimate Relationships, 46*(3), 351–71.

Kiecolt-Glaser, J., & Wilson, S. J. (2017). Lovesick: How Couples' Relationships Influence Health. *Annual Review of Clinical Psychology, May 8*(13), 421–43.

Krause. K. D. (2020). The Impact of Resilience on Health: Lessons Learned and Future Directions. *Behavioral Medicine, 46*(3/4), 375–78.

Kreager, D. (2008). Guarded Borders: Adolescent Interracial Romance and Peer Trouble at School. *Social Forces, 87*(2), 887–910.

Kroeger, R., & Williams, K. (2011). Consequences of Black Exceptionalism? Interracial Unions with Blacks, Depressive Symptoms, and Relationship Satisfaction. *The Sociological Quarterly, 52*, 400–20.

LaVeist, T. A. (2005). Disentangling Race and Socioeconomic Status: A Key to Understanding Health Inequalities. *Journal of Urban Health: Bulletin of the New York Academy of Medicine, 82*(2), iii26–iii34.

Lawton, B., Foeman, A., & Braz, M. (2012). Interracial Couples' Conflict Styles on Educational Issues. *Journal of Intercultural Communication Research, 42*(1), 35–53.

LeBlanc, A. J., Frost, D. M., & Wight, R. G. (2015). Minority Stress and Stress Proliferation Among Same-Sex and Other Marginalized Couples. *Journal of Marriage and Family, 77*(1), 40–59.

Lehmiller, J. J., & Agnew, C. R. (2006). Marginalized relationships: The impact of social disapproval on romantic relationship commitment. *Personality and Social Psychology Bulletin, 32*, 40–51.

Lewinsohn, P. M., Rohde, P., Seeley, J. R., Klein, D. N., & Gotlib, I. H. (2003). Psychosocial Functioning of Young Adults Who Have Experienced and Recovered from Major Depressive Disorder During Adolescence. *Journal of Abnormal Psychology, 112*(3), 353–63.

Lewis, R. Jr. (2014). Status of Interracial Marriage in the United States: A Qualitative Analysis of Interracial Spouse Perceptions. *International Journal of Social Science Studies, 2*(1), 16–25.

Link, B. G., & Phelan, J. C. (1995). Social Conditions as Fundamental Causes of Disease. *Journal of Health and Social Behavior, Extra Issue*, 80–94.

Link, B. G., & Phelan, J. C. (2001). Conceptualizing Stigma. *Annual Review of Sociology 27*, 363–85.

Lloyd, K. D., Katz, A. S., & Pronk, N. P. (2016). Building Emotional Resilience at the Workplace. *American College of Sports Medicine Health and Fitness Journal,* (January/February), 42–46. https://archive.hshsl.umaryland.edu/bitstream/handle/10713/13331/Building_Emotional_Resilience_at_the_Workplace__A.12.pdf?sequence=1&isAllowed=y.

Mann, M., Hosman, C. M. H., Schaalma, H. P., & de Vries, N. K. (2004). Self-esteem in a broad-spectrum approach for mental health promotion. *Health Education Research, 19*(4), 357–72.

Marmot M. (2003). Self-esteem and health. *BMJ (Clinical research ed.)*, 327(7415), 574–75.

Marquez-Velarde, G., Jones, N. E., & Keith, V. M. (2020). Racial stratification in self-rated health among Black Mexicans and White Mexicans. *SSM—Population Health, 10*, 1–8.

Martin, B., Cui, M., Ueno, K., & Fincham, F. D. (2013). Intimate Partner Violence in Interracial and Monoracial Couples. *Family Relations, 61*(1), 202–11.

Medlineplus.gov. (2021). *Stress and your health. MedlinePlus.* https://medlineplus.gov/ency/article/003211.htm.

Michaelson, J, Mahony, S., & Schifferes, J. (2012). Measuring Well-being: A guide for practitioners. *New Economics Foundations.* https://b.3cdn.net/nefoundation/8d92cf44e70b3d16e6_rgm6bpd3i.pdf.

Miller, B. (2014). What are the odds: An examination of adolescent interracial romance and risk for depression. *Youth & Society, 49*(2), 180–202.

Miller, B., James, A., & Roy, R. N. (2022). Loving Across Racial Lines: Associations between Gender and Partner Race and the Health of Young Adults. *Journal of Child and Family Studies, 31*(2), 703–15.

Miller, B., Rocks, S., Catalina, S., Zemaitis, N., Daniels, K., & Londono, J. (2019). The Missing Link in Contemporary Health Disparities Research: A Profile of the Mental and Self- Rated Health of Multiracial Young Adults. *Health Sociology Review, 28*(2), 209–27.

Miller, B., & Kail, B. L. (2016). Exploring the effects of spousal race on the self-rated health of intermarried adults. *Sociological Perspectives, 59*(3), 604–18.

Miller, B., Rote, S., & Keith, V. (2013). Coping with Racial Discrimination: Assessing the Vulnerability of African Americans and the Mediated Moderation of Psychosocial Resources. *Society and Mental Health, 3*(2), 133–50.

Miller, B., & Taylor, J. (2012). Racial and Socioeconomic Status Differences in Depressive Symptoms Among Black and White Youth: An Examination of the Mediating Effects of Family Structure, Stress and Support. Journal of Youth and Adolescence, 41,

Monk, Ellis P. Jr. (2015). The Cost of Color: Skin Color, Discrimination, and Health among African-Americans. *American Journal of Sociology, 121*(2), 396–444.

Monk, E. P. (2021). The Unceasing Significance of Colorism: Skin Tone Stratification in the United States. *Daedalus, 150*(2), 76–90.

Murray, S. L., Griffin, D., Rose, P., & Bellavia, G. (2006). For Better or Worse? Self-Esteem and the Contingencies of Acceptance in Marriage. *PSPB, 32*(7), 866–80.

NCCJ. (2021). *Colorism*. Retrieved May 1, 2020 (https://www.nccj.org/colorism-0).

Ozbay, F., Johnson, D. C., Dimaoulas, E., Morgan, C. A., Charney, D., & Southwick, S. (2007). Social Support and Resilience to Stress: From Neurobiology to Clinical Practice. *Psychiatry (Edgmont) 4*(5), 35–40.

Passel, J., Wang, W., & Taylor, P. (2010, June 4). Marrying Out: One-in-Seven New U.S. Marriages Is Interracial or Interethnic. *Pew Research Center's Social & Demographic Trends Project.* https://www.pewresearch.org/social-trends/2010/06/04/marrying-out/.

Pearlin, L. I. (1989). The Sociological Study of Stress. *Journal of Health and Social Behavior, 30*, 241–56.

Pearlin, L. I., Lieberman, M., Menaghan, E., & Mullan, J. (1981). *The Stress Process. Journal of Health and Social Behavior, 22*, 337–56.

Pearlin, L. I., & Schooler, C. (1978). The structure of coping. Journal of Health and Social Behavior, 19(1), 2–21. https://doi.org/10.2307/2136319.

Pew Research Center. (2017). *Intermarriage in the U.S. 50 Years After Loving v. Virginia.* http://www.pewsocialtrends.org/2017/05/18/intermarriage-in-the-u-s-50-years-after-loving-v-virginia/.

Phelan, J. C., Link, B. G., & Tehranifar, P. (2010). Social Conditions as Fundamental Causes of Health Inequalities: Theory, Evidence, and Policy Implications. *Journal of Health and Social Behavior, 51*(S), S28–S40.

Qian, Z., & Lichter, D. T. (2011). Changing patterns of interracial marriage in a multiracial society. Journal of Marriage and Family, 73(5), 1065–84.

Ramezankhan, A., Azizi, F., & Hadaegh, F. (2019). Associations of marital status with diabetes, hypertension, cardiovascular disease and all-cause mortality: A long term follow up studies. *PLoS ONE, 14(*4), 1–15.

Riggio, H. R., Weiser, D. A., Valenzuela, A. M., Lui, P., P., & Heuer, R. M. J. (2013). Self-Efficacy in Romantic Relationships: Prediction of Relationship Attitudes and Outcomes. *The Journal of Social Psychology, 153*(6), 629–50.

Robards, J., Evandrou, M., Falkingham, J., & Vlachantoni, A. (2012). Marital status, health and mortality. *Maturitas, 73*(4), 295–99.

Rosenthal, L., & Starks, T. J. (2015). Relationship Stigma and Relationship Outcomes in Interracial and Same-Sex Relationships: Examination of Sources and Buffers. *Journal of Family Psychology, 29*(6), 818–30.

Schipper, K., & Abma, T. A. (2011). Coping, family and mastery: top priorities for social science research bypatients with chronic kidney disease. *Nephrology Dialysis Transplantation, 26*, 3189–95.

Seshadri, G., & Knudson-Martin, C. (2013). How Couples Manage Interracial and Intercultural Differences: Implications for Clinical Practice. *Journal of Marital and Family Therapy, 39*(1), 43–58.

Shim, R. S., Ye, J., Baltrus, P., Fry-Johnson, Y., Daniels, E., & Rust, G. (2012). Racial/ethnic disparities, social support, and depression: examining a social determinant of mental health. *Ethnicity & Disease, 22*(1), 15–20.

Simon, R. W., & Barrett, A. E. (2010). Nonmarital Romantic Relationships and Mental Health in Emerging Adulthood: Does the Association Differ for Women and Men?. *Journal of Health and Social Behavior, 51*(2), 168–82.

Smith, K. P., & Christakis, N. A. (2008). Social Networks and Health. *Annual Review of Sociology, 34*, 405–29.

Smith, S., M., & Vale, W. W. (2006). The role of the hypothalamus-pituitary-adrenal axis in neuroendocrine responses to stress. *Dialogues of Clinical Neuroscience, 8*, 383–95.

Sohoni, D. (2007). Unsuitable Suitors: Anti-Miscegenation Laws, Naturalization Laws, and the Construction of Asian Identities. *Law & Society Review, 41*(3), 587–618.

Solsberry, P. W. (1994). Interracial Couples in the United State of America: Implications for Mental Health Counseling. *Journal of Mental Health Counseling, 16*(3), 304–17.

Sprecher, S., Brooks, J. E., Avogo, W. (2013). Self-Esteem Among Young Adults: Differences and Similarities Based on Gender, Race, and Cohort (1990–2012). *Sex Roles, 69*, 264–75.

Steinbugler, Amy. 2014. racial divides. *Contexts, 13*(2): 32–37.

Surtees, P. G., Wainwright, N. W. J., Luben, R., Wareham, N. J., Bingham, S. A., & Khaw, K.- T. (2010). Mastery is associated with cardiovascular disease mortality in men and women at apparently low risk. Health Psychology, 29(4), 412–20.

Symoens, S., Colman, E., & Bracke, P. (2014). Divorce, conflict, and mental health: how the quality of intimate relationships is linked to post-divorce well-being. *Journal of Applied Social Psychology, 44*, 220–23.

Thoits P. A. (1995). Stress, coping, and social support processes: where are we? What next? *Journal of Health and Social Behavior, Special*, 53–79.

Thoits, P. (2011). Mechanisms Linking Social Ties and Support to Physical and Mental Health. *Journal of Health and Social Behavior, 52*(2), 145–61.

Thomas, P.A., Liu, H., & Umberson, D. (2017). Family Relationships and Well-Being. *Innovation in Aging, 1*(3), 1–11.

Thompson, M. S., & Keith, V. M. (2001). The Blacker the Berry: Gender, Skin Tone, Self-Esteem, and Self-Efficacy. *Gender & Society, 15*(3), 336–57.

Tillman, K., & Miller, B. (2017). The role of family relationships in the psychological wellbeing of interracially dating adolescents. *Social Science Research, 65*, 240–52.

Tobin, C. S. T., Erving, C. L., & Barve, A. (2021). Race and SES Differences in Psychosocial Resources: Implication for Social Stress Theory. Social Psychology Quarterly, 84(1), 1–25.

Tran, A. G. & Lee, R. M. (2010). Perceived Ethnic-Racial Socialization, Ethnic Identity, and Social Competence Among Asian American Late Adolescents. *Cultural Diversity and Ethnic Minority Psychology, 15*(2), 169–78.

Tsay, S., & Chao, Y. (2002). Effects of perceived self-efficacy and functional status on depression in patients with chronic heart failure. *The Journal of Nursing Research, 10* (4), 271–78.

Turner, R. J. (2013). Understanding Health Disparities: The Relevance of Stress Process Model. *Society and Mental Health, 3*(3), 170–86.

Turner, R. J., & Marino, F. (1994). Social Support and Social Structure: A Descriptive Epidemiology. *Journal of Health and Social Behavior 35*(September):193–212.

Turner, R. J., & Turner, J. B. (1999). Social integration and support. In C. S. Aneshensel & J. C. Phelan (Eds.), Handbook of sociology of mental health (pp. 301–19). Kluwer Academic Publishers.

Turner, R. J., Brown, T., & Hale, W. B. (2017). Race, Socioeconomic Position, and Physical Health: A Descriptive Analysis. *Journal of Health and Social Behavior 58*(1): 23–36.

Turner, R. J., Wheaton, B., & Lloyd, D. (1995). The epidemiology of stress. *American Sociological Review, 60*, 104–25.

Tyndall, B.D., & C.A. Christie-Mizell. (2016) Mastery, Homeownership, and Adult Roles During the Transition to Adulthood. *Sociological Inquiry, 86*(1), 5–28.

Villazor, R. C. (2018). Residential Segregation and Interracial Marriages. *Fordham Law Review,86*, 2717–26. https://ir.lawnet.fordham.edu/4r/vol86/iss6/7.

Waite, L. J. (2018). Social Well-Being and Health in the Older Population: Moving beyond Social Relationships. In Hayward, M. D., & Majmundar, M. K. (Eds.), *Future Directions for the Demography of Aging: Proceedings of a Workshop* (pp. 99–130). The National Academies Press.

Waite, L., & Gallagher, M. (2000). *The Case for Marriage: Why Married People are Happier, Healthier, and Better Off Financially*. Broadway Books.

Wang, H., Kao, G., & Joyner, K. (2006). Stability of interracial and intraracial romantic relationships among adolescents. *Social Science Research, 35*, 435–53.

Wang, W. (2012, February 16). The Rise of Intermarriage: Rates, Characteristics Vary by Race and Gender. Pew Research Center. https://www.pewresearch.org/social-trends/2012/02/16/the-rise-of-intermarriage/.

Weiser, D. A., & Weigel, D. J. (2016). Self-efficacy in romantic relationships: Direct and indirect effects on relationship maintenance and satisfaction. *Personality and Individual Differences, 89*, 152–156. https://doi.org/10.1016/j.paid.2015.10.013.

Weisskirch, R. S. (2017). Abilities in romantic relationships and well-being among emerging adults. *Marriage & Family Review 53*(1), 36–47.

Winefield, H. R., Gill, T. K., Taylor, A. W., & Pilkington, R. M. (2012). Psychological well-being and psychological distress: is it necessary to measure both? *Psychology of Well-Being 2*(3): 1–14. https://psywb.springeropen.com/track/pdf/10.1186/2211-1522-2-3.pdf.

Williams, D. R., & Collins, C. (1995). US Socioeconomic and Racial Differences in Health: Patterns and Explanations. *Annual Review of Sociology, 21*, 349–86.

Williams, D. R., Lawrence, J. A., & Davis, B. A. (2019). Racism and Health: Evidence and Needed Research. *Annual Review of Public Health, 40*, 105–25.

Williams, D. R., & Williams-Morris, R. (2000). Racism and mental health: the African American experience. *Ethnicity & health 5*(3/4): 243–68. doi:10.1080/713667453.

Wilson, S. E. (2001). Socioeconomic Status and the Prevalence of Health Problems Among Married Couples in Late Midlife. *American Journal of Public Health, 90*(1), 131–35.

Wong, J. S., & Penner, A. M. (2018). Better Together? Interracial Relationships and Depressive Symptoms. *Socius: Sociological Research for a Dynamic World, 4*, 1–11.

World Health Organization. (1948). *Preamble to the Constitution of the World Health Organization as adopted by the International Health Conference*, New York, 19–22 June 1946; signed on 22 July 1946 by the representatives of sixty-one states (Official Records of the World Health Organization, no. 2, p. 100) and entered into force on 7 April 1948. /3/2015/06/ST_15.06.11_MultiRacial-Timeline.pdf.

Wright, K. (2016). Social Networks, Interpersonal Social Support, and Health Outcomes: A Health Communication Perspective. *Frontiers in Communication, 1*(10), 1–6.

Yancey, G. (2007). Experiencing Racism: Differences in the Experiences of Whites Married to Blacks and Non-Black Racial Minorities. *Journal of Comparative Family Studies, 38*(2), 197–213.

Youssef, N. A., Belew, D., Hao, G., Wang, X., Treiber, F. A., Stefanek, M., Yassa, M., Boswell, E., McCall, W. V., & Su, S. (2017). Racial/ethnic differences in the association of childhood adversities with depression and the role of resilience. *Journal of Affective Disorders, January 15*(208), 577–81.

Yu, Y., & Zhang, Z. (2017). Interracial Marriage and Self-Reported Health of Whites and Blacks in the United States. *Population Research and Policy Review*, 36(6), 851–70.

Zalta, A. K., & Chambless, D. L. (2012). Understanding gender differences in anxiety: The mediating effects of instrumentality and mastery. Psychology of Women Quarterly, 36(4), 488–99.

Chapter 4

Bridging Family and Friends

CHAPTER OVERVIEW

As primary agents of socialization, the beliefs and behaviors of a person's family and friends tend to have a major impact on the lives and well-being of young adults (Giddens et al., 2019). For many people, family members establish initial boundaries as for who is and is not considered an acceptable partner (Bell & Hastings, 2015; Edmonds & Killen, 2009), and friendship networks often provide opportunities for romantic involvement as well as reification of a partner's acceptability (Clark-Ibanez & Femlee, 2004; Kao, Joyner, & Balistreri, 2019). However, the socio-demographic (e.g., race, gender, ages, and socioeconomic status) background of a person's family and friends tend to have extensive effects on an individual's racial socialization, views on race and race relations, exposure to other-race groups, and perceived acceptability of romantic involvement within and across racial groups.

For many young adults, the race of one's partner is strongly tied to their perceived approval from family and friends, which can be problematic since 10 percent of adults (over twenty-five million people) disapprove of interracial romance among their own family members, including 5 percent of young adults ages 18 to 29 (Pew Research Center, 2017). Given that stigmatized statuses like race and interracial relationships are considered social stressors (Goffman, 1963; Miller, 2014), it is likely that young adults in IRRs can experience a unique type of double jeopardy whereby they are exposed to social stressors related to their relationship *and* they lose the support of family and friends that disapprove of interracial partnerships. Consequently, young adults in interracial relationships (IRRs), especially those not conforming to family and friends' norms of racial homogamy, are likely to face stressors that increase their vulnerability to poorer health outcomes more than those in same-race relationships (SRRs).

From this perspective, understanding the health of the Bridge Kids and other interracially involved persons requires exploring the impact their social network of family and friends has on their health. It is therefore the goal of this chapter to explore the impact family and friends have on the lives and well-being of the Bridge Kids and others in IRRs. In particular, the discussion focuses on how socialization from family and friends shape the race a person chooses for their partner in the assortative mating process, the way partner's race impacts relationships within one's social network, and how these determinants effect the health of those in interracial romantic relationships.

RACIAL SOCIALIZATION

Socialization is the lifelong process whereby people learn the behaviors that are expected and acceptable within society (Giddens et al., 2019). The complex socialization process in diverse societies like the United States includes the conscious and unconscious behaviors and attitudes people learn from other social agents such as family, peers, work, the media and social institutions (Giddens et al., 2019; Link, 2009). Family and friends are usually people's most influential agents of socialization, however, because they play a critical role in shaping an individual's beliefs and actions, especially for young adults like the Bridge Kids.

In racially diverse societies, racial socialization is one specific form of socialization scholars investigate to better understand the effect of race and race relations. *Racial socialization* refers to learning the beliefs and practices regarding racial status, group identity, and intergroup relationships that are conveyed within socially stratified and racially diverse societies (Tran & Lee, 2010). Overall, racial socialization aims to teach people the numerous ways race impacts their lives in the systemic process of the developing their self-identity and social identity, as well as how to potentially handle issues and experiences related to racism and racial discrimination (Hughes et al., 2009; Hughes et al., 2017).

Mainstream perceptions of racial groups vary widely in the United States, however, as members of some Asian groups (e.g., Chinese, Japanese, and South Korean) are referred to as *model minorities* and *honorary Whites* whereas other Asian groups (e.g., Laotian and Hmong) and Blacks receive much less deference than other groups (Lee & Bean 2004; Shih et al., 2019). Accordingly, some families address race-based issues by socializing young adults about differences in racial identities so that they learn about racism, prejudice, discrimination, and privilege (Hughes et al., 2017; Neblett et al., 2009). Parents and other family members engage in the racial socialization process in a variety of ways including openly discussing race and race-based issues, downplaying the importance of race, and avoiding the topic of race altogether (Hagerman, 2014; Hughes et al., 2006; Neblett et al., 2009).

The rationale for, and types of, racial socialization to which people are subjected to can greatly differ by their family. For example, some immigrants choose to reside in ethnic enclaves that minimize their exposure to discriminatory behaviors while allowing for the preservation of their own cultural heritage (Rong & Fitchett, 2008). Other strategies include Black and Hispanic families socializing their children on how to recognize and deal with the different types of prejudice they are likely to encounter (Hughes et al., 2017; Tran & Lee, 2010). Racial minority parents' own experiences with discrimination in childhood, at work, and in their daily lives also impacts how they socialize their children on what to expect and how to cope with racial discrimination, especially from White persons (White-Johnson, Ford & Sellers, 2010). As such, experiences of racism and discrimination are likely to vary within and between racial groups, as well as the messages about racial socialization conveyed by families.

It also seems reasonable to assume that racial socialization significantly influences an individual's attitudes toward interracial romance. Beginning in childhood, family and friends greatly influence the development of a person's beliefs and behaviors about race and racial interactions (James et al., 2018). The attitudes and actions of family and friends can significantly affect young people's opportunities and willingness to develop friendships and romantic relationships that cross racial lines. For example, Wieling (2003) found that attitudes towards the acceptance of interracial romance vary by the race of one's partner as some White and Hispanic young adults in IRRs said that if their partner "had been Black, that would have been a whole other story" (p. 51). This sentiment implies the family and friends of White and Hispanic persons may be less accepting of them being in an IRR with a Black partner, a finding that supports nationally representative survey data showing people are least accepting of family members being interracially married to a Black partner (Passel et al., 2010). In other words, family and friends' approval of a person's IRR vary by the couple's racial composition (e.g., White-Hispanic, or Black-Hispanic). Through the racial socialization process, young people learn why people support or oppose IRRs, as well as how their own interracial involvement may affect, or be affected by, their family and friends.

BRIDGE KIDS' FAMILIES

Whether in a manner that is negative or positive, family members are often the most influential people in the lives of the Bridge Kids and others in IRRs. Families are complex and diverse social networks consisting of a person's siblings, parents, grandparents, and extended kin, all of whom may directly and indirectly express their opinions about the acceptability of romantic partnerships (Bell & Hastings, 2015; Miller et al., 2021). A family's beliefs towards IRRs are especially important to the Bridge Kids since persons ages 18 to 29 are least likely to oppose if a close relative intermarries (Pew Research Center, 2017) and most likely to be interracially involved themselves (Jones, 2005). Nearly two-thirds of Americans (63 percent) express being fine if a family member were to intermarry, but 37 percent say they will be bothered or not at all accepting of an intermarried family member (Passel et al., 2010). This means that for people in IRRs, family members that accept their mixed-race relationship may be sources of social support whereas those that oppose may be sources of social strain or stressors.

Family members can project their support for interracial romance in numerous ways. By engaging in IRRs themselves, family members show strong support for interracial romance. At present, more than one-third (35% percent) of American adults have a close family member who has been intermarried (Passel et al., 2010) and countless more have relatives in nonmarital interracial partnerships. This suggests that over seventy million Americans have at least one close family member in an IRR (infoplease.com, 2020), which signals to the younger and more impressionable kin that their family approves of interracial romance. Family support of interracial romance can also be directly conveyed to their kinship. For example, after disclosing her interracial involvement to her parents, a Black female with a White boyfriend expresses how her family supports her decision by stating that "[t]hey were very positive about it. . . . My family is understanding and accepting" (Bell & Hastings, 2015; p. 764). Such support is surely meaningful to the well-being of those in IRRs.

In contrast, family members can also directly or indirectly express their opposition to interracial involvement. For instance, a White female recalls her father explicitly telling her "If you ever bring home a black guy, don't expect to have this as your home or me as your father!" (Prather, 1990; p. 152), which exemplifies how family can influence the interracial partner selection process by deterring interracial involvement while also being sources of social strain for those in IRRs. Similarly, another White female recalls the anger she faced after telling her family about her Black boyfriend as she stated, "One day, my mom called me and said, 'Who is this Jack guy, what are you doing, what is going on? Is he Black?' and I said, 'Yes and it really does not matter to me.' She said, 'You know how your father is going to feel about this, what are you thinking?' Then my dad got on the phone and said, 'you stupid little bitch'" (Bell & Hastings, 2015, p. 762). This example points to the expectations some families have for conformity and not independent thoughts or actions in terms of assortative mating. Like theses fathers, relatives voice their points of view about expected relationship behavior as well as the informal sanctions that may be imposed upon family members who do not conform to those expectations (Edmonds & Killen, 2009), which is especially relevant to those family members that become interracially involved even against family opposition.

Perceptions of family as sources of social support or social strain is particularly salient for the health of individuals in mixed-race relationships. Family social support is positively associated with numerous health outcomes (Miller & Taylor, 2012; Thoits, 2011; Tillman & Miller, 2017; Thomas, Liu, & Umberson, 2017), indicating that people who perceive their family is supportive of their IRR are likely to have better health than those that do not have the support of their family. Conversely, young adults and others who engage in interracial relationships without the approval of their parents may experience intensively negative parental reactions, elevated parent-child conflict (Bell & Hastings, 2015; Downey et al., 1999; McNamara et al., 1999; Yahya & Boag, 2014), and risk losing their primary source of social support (Laursen & Jensen-Campbell, 1999). As a result, people in interracial romantic relationships may face a unique type of *double jeopardy* (Ferraro and Farmer, 1996; Mendelson et al., 2008), which increases their risk of having poor health due to experiencing elevated levels of stress because of the stigma and negative reactions associated with their relationship choice, while also perceiving lower levels of the kinds of social support needed to protect their well-being in the face elevated levels of stress. Individuals in IRRs may therefore have poorer health than those in SRRs, due to the cumulative effects of their increased social strains and stressors that is offset by a decrease in the social support they need to help them cope with the deleterious effects of those stressors. As a result, for interracially partnered individuals, family social support is beneficial to their health but the social strain from unsupportive family is harmful.

Much of the current literature examining whether family supports or opposes IRRs tends to focus on the "family" as a whole (Jones, 2005; Newport, 2013; Passel et al., 2010), and much less is known about how a person's choice to be interracially involved is associated with the attitudes or expectations of specific family members (e.g., siblings, parents, grandparents). At present, we do know that young adults like the Bridge Kids are much more likely to be interracially involved if they believe their siblings, parents, and grandparents will accept their decision to date outside their racial group (Miller et al., 2021; Yahya & Boag, 2014). The likelihood for interracial romance among the Bridge Kids is greatest when they perceive their siblings would approve, followed by parents, then grandparents (Miller et al., 2021). Approval of a family member being interracially involved is also strongly correlated with age, with the youngest family members expressing the greater acceptance of interracial romance and the oldest voicing the greatest opposition (Pew Research Center, 2017). Based on the existing data, it seems reasonable to hypothesize that the notion of a family member's acceptance of interracial romance is generally strongest among the youngest generations and weakest among the oldest.

Family Systems Theory suggests that examining the dynamics of different family relationships is generally important because families are not one unified system, but rather organized into interdependent, reciprocally influential subsystems. These subsystems are composed of distinct relationships between parents and children, between siblings, between grandparents and grandchildren, and so forth (Whiteman, McHale, & Soli, 2011). Moreover, it is especially crucial to account for differences in race, race relations, and racial socialization when considering the impact of one's family on their involvement in interracial relationships. From this perspective the reframed Family Systems Theory, which incorporates the roles race and racism play in accounting for differences in family experiences (James et al., 2018), can help us better understand the differential influences family subsystems have on the interracial partner selection process and the lives of those that are interracially involved (Miller, 2020). The following sections therefore use the overarching perspective of the reframed Family Systems Theory to discuss the impact family subsystems have on the interracial partner selection process and well-being of young adults, beginning with the youngest likely group to have close kinship ties with the Bridge Kids, their siblings.

BRIDGE KIDS' SIBLINGS

Most young adults in the United States grow up with at least one sister or brother (Milevsky, 2011), which plays an instrumental role in their socialization process (Kramer et al. 2019). Siblings help their brothers and sisters learn broader social expectations, as well as the behaviors and beliefs specific to his or her family. Because of their shared social environments and family experiences, siblings are also an important part of the racial socialization process and often hold similar views on topics such as race and race relations (Doughty, McHale, & Feinberg, 2015; Stocker, Burwell, & Briggs, 2002).

Sibling relationships have various functions that are distinct from interactions with their parents and other family members. Depending on the family's circumstances (e.g., working parents, foster care, deceased parent, cultural expectations, blended families, etc.), older siblings may serve as caregivers or de facto parents (Kramer et al., 2019), which makes them very influential over the decision making of their younger brothers and sisters. Moreover, when it comes to their own romantic relationships, young adults often feel more comfortable discussing issues related to romance and intimacy with their siblings than their parents (Kowal & Blinn-Pike, 2004). In such instances, siblings also serve as confidants, sources of social support, and advisors to one another (Killoren & Roach, 2014; Tucker, McHale, & Crouter, 2001). Siblings can therefore be very influential in the partner selection process, especially in terms of shaping one another's beliefs and behaviors about romantic relationships that are very different than other family members.

Not surprisingly, siblings can be very influential in the partner selection process especially in terms of shaping one another's beliefs and behaviors about romantic relationships generally, and interracial romance specifically. For one, the attitudes and social networks of a person's sibling may help facilitate the formation of romantic relationships, as people sometimes meet potential partners through their brothers and sisters. Siblings with racially diverse networks may not only provide connections to potential partners of differing racial backgrounds, but they are also more likely to approve of interracial romance or even be interracially involved themselves (Kreager, 2008; Wang, Kao, & Joyner, 2006). Accordingly, like other family members, siblings in IRRs act as examples for their beliefs on the acceptability of such relationships.

On one hand, a person may see their sibling(s) in same-race relationships and presume that is what they are expected to do as well. Conversely, a young adult may see their sibling in an interracial relationship and perceive that such relationships are deemed okay by their sibling (Pryor, 2018). Siblings can also clash over who is viewed as an appropriate partner if one sibling stepped outside of the family norm of forming same-race relationships. However, instead of causing conflict, it is also possible that having a brother or sister in an IRR may actually establish a precedent for their other sibling(s) to follow regarding the acceptability of crossing racial lines for romance.

It is in this manner that an individual's deidentification can also play a role in a sibling's decision to become interracially involved, especially when considering the influence older siblings have on their brothers and sisters (Kramer et al., 2019). *Deidentification* is the process whereby "individual siblings may differentiate themselves and establish their own unique identity, role, or niche within the family system; this identity is shaped, in part, by that individual's perceptions of their siblings' identities" (Kramer et al., 2019; p. 2). Deidentification can be associated with the partner selection process of young adults in that, for example, a young man might observe his older brother in a same-race relationship and intentionally choose to date interracially to differentiate himself from his brother.

There are numerous ways that siblings may significantly impact the health of their interracially involved brothers and/or sisters. Siblings that do not conform to the expected family norms and become interracially involved, may experience conflict in the relationships with their brothers and sisters. For instance, regarding his siblings' reaction towards his cross-cultural relationship, an Australian Jewish male with a non-Jewish girlfriend stated that "my mum loves her, but my older brother finds it difficult" (Yahya & Boag, 2014; p. 765). This statement highlights that crossing racial lines for romance may become a source of social strain and conflict between siblings that can result in a loss of support from one's brothers and sisters (Killoren & Roach, 2014; Tucker, McHale, & Crouter, 2001). Conversely, siblings can serve as confidants who support their brothers and sisters in IRRs by introducing them to their other-race friends or even being in interracial relationships themselves. Therefore, having brothers and sisters that oppose IRRs are likely sources of stress that adversely impact one's health, whereas having siblings who are accepting of interracial romance, especially those in IRRs themselves, are likely to be sources of social support that benefit the well-being of the Bridge Kids and others in IRRs.

BRIDGE KIDS' PARENTS

The relationship between parents and their children is perhaps the most impactful subsystem in family dynamics, especially for molding their children's attitudes and actions concerning the interracial partner selection process (Laursen & Jensen-Campbell, 1999; Okitikpi, 2009). For young adults, parents often set the tone for the characteristics and partners with whom their children become romantically involved. This means establishing a pool of acceptable romantic partners, boundaries for appropriate dating behaviors, and sanctions for involvement with persons considered to be unacceptable partners (Edmonds & Killen, 2009; Laursen & Jensen-Campbell, 1999). For many parents, however, the race of their child's partner is an important characteristic that influences their notions of partner acceptability (Edmonds & Killen, 2009; Laursen & Jensen-Campbell, 1999). Consequently, the socialization of parents plays a crucial role in determining whether or not their children are willing and able to engage in IRRs.

It should be noted that we cannot overlook the growing number of parents that are in interracial relationships themselves. For some parents in IRRs, the partnership itself should acknowledge to their children that they approve of interracial romance (Doucet, Hall, & Giraud, 2019). In turn, young adults raised in Multiracial families with interracial parents may view IRRs as normative and thus become more likely to engage in an IRR themselves. Conversely, since many interracially involved people report experiencing various forms of prejudice and racial discrimination associated with their relationship in social spaces as well as from their families (Steinbugler, 2012;

van der Walt & Basson, 2015), it is possible that parents in IRRs may discourage their children from becoming interracially involved because of their own experiences from being in a socially marginalized relationship.

It should go without saying that some parents are quite critical of IRRs (Miller et al., 2004), and directly express this disapproval to their children as an attempt to deter or restrict them from being interracially involved (Bell & Hastings, 2015; Edmonds & Killen, 2009). Many young adults internalize the beliefs of their parents whom they do not want to disrespect or displease, so they parrot their parent's opposition to interracial romance like an Asian male who stated, "My parents, just as most Korean parents that I have contact with, banish the idea of interracial dating" (Clark-Ibanez & Femlee, 2004, pp. 300). A Hispanic female similarly said, "It would be hard [to date inter-ethnically] because my parents wouldn't agree with it and neither would my [H]ispanic friends. They've all told me not to mix blood. Stay with your own" (Clark-Ibanez & Femlee, 2004, p. 300). Such statements clearly demonstrate that some parents definitely socialize their children to eschew any interracial romantic involvement.

The belief in "mixing blood" is especially interesting because it highlights the idea that some people view race in terms of genetics and therefore view interracial relationships as deplorable for blending genetically disparate racial groups. This perspective is shared by a White male who stated his interracial relationship with a Black female:

> really breaks [his mother's] heart, when she starts thinking about what my children would look like if Nikole and I get married. I have blond hair and blue eyes and my mother does also. I get compliments on how I look like my mother. It breaks her heart that our future kids won't be blond-haired and blue-eyed. The last time she and I spoke explicitly about interracial relationships, we both cried . . . and it really hurt. For my mother, skin color made a difference (Bell & Hastings, 2015: pp. 763).

In another example, after telling her mother about her intentions to marry a Black man, one White mother bluntly told her daughter, "Not just because he's Black, he could have been Hispanic, he could have been Japanese, Vietnamese, people should stay with their own, you should stick with your own kind . . . whites should stay with whites, Blacks should stay with Blacks, Chinese should stay with Chinese, and Indians should stay with Indians. . . . I just don't think you should mix cultures and mix colors [or] ethnicities" (Pryor, 2018; pp. 109–10). Sadly, and consequently, such parental beliefs and behaviors have led many people in IRRs to believe that their parents disapprove of their relationships, hold racist attitudes, pressure them to uphold their cultures (Yahya & Boag, 2014), and are worried about the possibility of mixed-race grandchildren (Morales, 2012).

Still, many people perceive one or both of their parents are very supportive of them being in an interracial relationship (Bell & Hastings, 2015). Not surprisingly, young adults like the Bridge Kids are 26 percent more likely to be in an IRR when they perceive their parents approve of interracial romance (Miller et al., 2021). It can be argued that parents who support their children in IRRs probably espouse a color-blind perspective where they racially socialize their children to believe people are all humans so racial identity does not matter (Rollins, 2019). As a White female remembers when her brother told her mother and grandmother, "I mean, you know, I'm in love with this girl [and] she is black. And they basically said, if you are happy, we are happy, we are not crazy about it, but we are not going to, by any means, disown you" (Pryor, 2018; p. 109). Such an open-minded mentality toward racial identity and interracial romance strongly reflects the use of one's sociological imagination in examining this issue. It therefore stands to reason those parents with color-blind beliefs could be more accepting of their children engaging in interracial romance.

Of particular interest is the fact that interracially involved young adults tend to have parents with a much more racially diverse network of friends than young adults that never dated interracially (Clark-Ibanez & Femlee, 2004). This suggests that parents who cross racial lines for friendships are probably more likely to accept, and maybe even support, their children crossing racial lines for romance. It also stands to reason that managing close social interactions with other-race people is part of the racial socialization Bridge Kids grow up learning from their parents. Perhaps even more than words or perceptions, seeing the true actions of how their parents approach race relations may be what matters most to young adults because mothers and fathers act as role models who demonstrate whether close relationships with those from different racial groups is acceptable.

Not all parents are so impartial to having other-race friends themselves or their children being in IRRs, which can have a severely negative impact on the well-being of the Bridge Kids and others in IRRs. Such pessimism, has led to some people in IRRs hearing their parents say things like, "You have to pick me or this White girl" (Bell & Hastings, 2015; p. 763). Those that do become interracially involved, however, report experiencing greater conflict and less close relationships with their parents (Dowdy & Kliewer, 1998; Joyner & Udry, 2000; Tillman & Miller, 2017). As a result, interracially involved young adults may be less able to rely on their parents to provide adequate social support because they perceive their parents are less caring and not as emotionally supportive (Tillman & Miller, 2017), which increases their vulnerability to poor health outcomes.

BRIDGE KIDS' GRANDPARENTS

As the parents of one's parents, the grandparent-grandchild relationship is extremely special in the family subsystem. Today, an increasing number of grandparents are taking on regular childrearing responsibilities for their grandchildren by either raising them independently or assisting their adult children on a day-to-day basis (Hayslip et al., 2013). Actively participating in the childrearing process and having a generally high social status in the family helps make many grandparents very influential in the socialization of their grandchildren. It is therefore very fitting that, like other family members, grandparents play a critical role in affecting the partner selection process and well-being outcomes of their grandchildren.

Considering that the average age of today's first-time grandparents is fifty years old (AARP.org, 2019) and the Bridge Kids are ages thirteen to twenty-nine, it seems fair to assume that most Bridge Kids have grandparents who are at least sixty-five years old. This is a unique juxtaposition in age groups given that the Bridge Kids are the most likely to be in an IRR and their grandparents, people sixty-five and older, are most likely to disapprove of a family member being interracially involved (Pew Research Center, 2017; Wang, 2012). The opposition some grandparents have towards interracial relationships may be related to their own experiences when race relations were extremely contentious during the Jim Crow era, when racial segregation and anti-miscegenation laws were both legal in many parts of the United States (Browning, 1951). Consequently, young adults that do cross racial lines for romance may cause conflict or strain in the relationships they have with their grandparents who might still view IRRs as taboo.

The oppositional attitudes toward interracial romance between many grandparents and their grandchildren undoubtedly contribute to college-aged students perceiving their grandparents as racists who strongly disapprove of mixed-race relationships (Yahya & Boag, 2014). Accordingly, some young adults feel it is difficult to "date someone of another ethnicity. Not because of any prejudices [they] have but because [they] come from family that doesn't approve of that. [Some] grandparents (on both sides) look down on dating other races" (Clark-Ibanez & Femlee, 2004: p. 300).

Besides being antagonists to IRRs, there are many elder persons that are, or have been, intermarried or in interracial relationships themselves. In fact, more than one in four (28 percent) of those ages sixty-five and over have interracially dated at least once in their life (Jones, 2005). The number of older adults in IRRs is also increasing as the proportion of intermarried newlyweds ages fifty and over has nearly tripled, from 5 percent in 1980 to 13 percent in 2015 (Pew Research Center, 2017). This group of grandparents with experience being in a in mixed-race relationships assuredly serve as examples for the acceptability of interracial romance to other family members, especially their grandchildren like the Bridge Kids.

In addition to those with experience being in an IRR, there are plenty of elderly adults that support interracial romance, believe IRRs are good for society, and approve of a family member being intermarried (Pew Research Center, 2017). The support from these grandparents has a tremendous impact on young adults like the Bridge Kids who are 23 percent more likely to be in an IRR when they perceive their grandparents approve of interracial romance, and White young adults are less willing to engage in interracial romance if they feel their grandparents would not approve (Miller et al., 2021). It is also important to note that many grandparents from racial minority groups support and encourage interracial romance because they see it as a means of their family's successful assimilation into mainstream society (Gordon, 1964). For instance, members of some Hispanic families are encouraged to intermarry with Whites so that subsequent generations will have a fair skin-tone that allows them to be seen as Hispanic but *White passing* so they gain all the benefits that *whiteness* provides (Killian, 2001; Stephens & Fernandez, 2012; Vasquez, 2015). Thus, the approval and social support of grandparents for their grandchildren in IRRs likely bolsters the quality of those grandparent-grandchild relationship, and it is probably beneficial to the well-being of interracially involved persons.

BRIDGE KIDS' EXTENDED KIN

The influence of extended kin in the partner selection process of young adults can be very important but is sometimes overlooked. Extended kin networks consist of an individual's aunts, uncles, cousins, and grandparents (Giddens et al., 2019), all of whom can be very influential agents of socialization in a person's life depending on the strength of their bonds and sphere of influence. Because they can be so robust and dynamic, the ability of these family members to effect one's socialization and partner selection processes can vary by the member's age, closeness of their relationships, network size, and frequency of contact between a person and their extended kin.

An attribute of a person's kinship network that is salient for the interracial partner selection process is the racial composition of their extended family. Given that one-third of Americans have family members in IRRs (Pew Research Center, 2017), and many of whom have Multiracial children (Pew research Center, 2015; Roy & Rollins, 2019) means more and more people are being exposed to, and interacting with, members of different racial groups. In fact, young adults with five or more interracially involved relatives are more than twice as likely to be in an IRR than those with no family members in IRRs (Miller et al., 2021). Therefore, the more interracially involved relatives a young adult has, the greater the likelihood he or she will be in an IRR themselves.

Those same interracially involved family are also probably supportive of other family members being in IRRs as well. Some interracially partnered couples acknowledge the acceptance and support they receive from their extended family (Pryor, 2018). This is important for individuals in IRRs that need to cope with chronic strains and stigma of interracial romance that those in SRRs do not face. Social support from family is therefore an especially important coping resource for people in IRRs because greater perceived family support is associated with better health outcomes (Miller & Taylor, 2012; Woods et al., 2019), particularly among romantically involved young adults (Tillman & Miller, 2017).

Although most people approve of intermarriage among family members, more than one-third of adults do not (Passel et al., 2010), which may result in awkward or strained social interactions between persons in IRRs and those extended family members that oppose such relationships. Because negative interactions with extended family is associated with lower romantic relationship satisfaction (Taylor et al., 2012), interracial couples may avoid, or disassociate themselves from, disapproving family members to elude the potential social strain. Additionally, not only is lower romantic relationship satisfaction is associated with worse physical, mental, and emotional well-being (Barr & Simons, 2014), but strained relationships with extended family may be more harmful to a person's health than relationship dissatisfaction (Woods et al., 2019). Therefore, the quality of a person's relationship with their extended kinship network can have a very strong influence on their assortative mating process and well-being, particularly for those that cross racial lines for romance.

BRIDGE KIDS' FRIENDS

Like family, friends are primary agents of socialization and important members of most people's social network. Friends are particularly important in the lives of young adults because they are the people with whom a person shares a bond of mutual affection (Merriam-Webster.com, 2021), and those closest of friends who are viewed and treated as if they were family are referred to as *fictive kin* (Giddens et al., 2019). Socially interacting with peers facilitates the personal development of young adults as they transition to spending much more free time with friends than their parents (Furman & Shaffer, 2003). Due to changing racial demographics, decreasing racial segregation in

U.S. neighborhoods, school integration, and social media (Iceland & Wilkes, 2006; Williams & Collins, 1995; Buggs, 2019), today's young adults have more opportunities than any previous generation to socially interact with, and befriend, others from different racial backgrounds than their own. Young adults' friendship networks also provide them with access to potential romantic partners as well as govern many of the social norms related to the partner selection process (Collins, 2003; Feiring, 1999; Laursen & Jensen-Campbell, 1999). Therefore, whether fictive kin or close companions, friends play a very important role in the assortative mating process of young adults, particularly for shaping a person's beliefs and behaviors about interracial romance.

The majority of young adults approve of IRRs, but about 5 percent of those ages 18 to 29 do not approve of intermarriage, and 5 percent also believe intermarriage is generally a bad thing for society (Pew Research Center, 2017). This means millions of young adults have friends that disapprove of IRRs. Peers often pressure one another to conform to group expectations regarding romantic involvement (Clark-Ibanez & Femlee, 2004; Connolly & Goldberg, 1999), so a young adult's choice to date interracially may oppose peer expectations of same-race romantic partnerships. For those in IRRs, the lack of peer conformity can potentially increase an individual's conflict with their friends and lessen perceptions of friends being emotionally supportive. Both conflict with friends and perceiving they are not supportive are associated with greater anxiety, greater depression, greater psychological distress, and lower life satisfaction (Brown et al., 2000; Daley & Hammen, 2002; Kessler et al., 1999; Prelow et al., 2006; Wight, Boticelli, & Aneshensel, 2006). Consequently, being in an IRR and having friends that disapprove of such relationships is probably very troubling and mentally challenging for interracially partnered individuals like the Bridge Kids and others.

Since interracial relationships remain socially marginalized and still are not universally accepted, young adults and others in IRRs are likely to be distressed by the negative social pressure, stigma, and discriminatory treatment they experience (Brooks & Lynch, 2019; Seshadri & Knudson-Martin, 2013; Solsberry, 1994). Knowing their relationships are stigmatized contributes to some young adults in IRRs perceiving more trouble from their peers (Kreager, 2008) and being less likely to publicly display affections towards their romantic partner than those with same-race partners (Vaquera & Kao, 2005). Such negative perceptions and reserved social behaviors probably add to the instability of IRRs and their increased possibility of dissolving sooner than same-race partnerships (Bratter & King, 2008; Wang, Kao, & Joyner, 2006; Zhang & Van Hook, 2014). This is a particularly concerning health issue because a romantic breakup increases a young adults' risk for depression among young adults (Barrett & Simon, 2010; Miller, 2014).

Despite the conflict and lack of support some people in IRRs experience with their friends, their peers are largely very accepting of interracial romance. About 95 percent of young adults approve of interracial marriage and 54 percent believe IRRs are good for society (Pew Research Center, 2017), suggesting most interracially involved young adults have friends that support them and approve of their relationship. Accordingly, one factor that influences the social support people in IRRs perceive from their friends is network size. In general, romantically involved youth tend to have more friends than their non-dating peers (Connolly et al., 2006; Kuttler & LaGreca, 2004) and those with larger friendship networks are less distressed than those with fewer friends (Falci & McNeely, 2009; LaGreca & Mackey, 2007). Having too many friends can also be problematic, however, as depressive symptoms have been shown to increase when the network size rises above a dozen or so friends (Falci & McNeely, 2009), which is probably due to the greater influence of each individual friend when the size of a person's network is smaller whereas the impact of each individual friend is lessened in larger networks (Giddens et al., 2019).

From within their peer networks, romantically involved adolescents report feeling more social support, greater social acceptance, and having less conflict with their close friends than do their non-dating peers (Wright et al., 2006; Kuttler & LaGreca, 2004; LaGreca & Lopez, 1998). Not surprisingly, perceiving high levels of support from friends is associated with having fewer depressive symptoms than those who believe their friends are not so supportive (Bovier et al., 2004; Gore & Aseltine, 2003; Needham, 2008). Thus, regardless if someone is in a SRR or IRR, romantically involved young adults probably experience better psychological well-being than their single because they tend to perceive having more social support from their relatively larger friendship networks (Kuttler & LaGreca, 2004), which may be especially beneficial to those in IRRs.

Besides having a relatively large group of friends, the racial diversity of one's friendship network is particularly salient to those in mixed-race relationships. Friendship networks not only provide social connections to potential romantic partners, but they also establish many of the social norms that regulate a young person's choice of partner (Kao et al., 2019; Laursen & Jensen-Campbell, 1999). Not surprisingly, most young adults become romantically involved with people within their friendship networks and do so, at least in part, based on the actual or perceived reactions from peers (Clark-Ibanez & Felmlee, 2004; Collins, 2003; Kao et al., 2019). As such, the racial composition of an individual's friendship network is therefore especially important because it can be very influential in shaping their attitudes towards race and race relations, as well as providing opportunities to engage in interracial romance. For these reasons, the racial diversity of a person's friendship network significantly influences their likelihood of dating inter-racially, as well as their friends' attitudes towards interracial partnerships.

In support of this premise, the *Intergroup Contact Hypothesis* posits that cross-racial contact is particularly valuable for interracial romantic rela-tionship formation because *individuals in interracial relationships tend to view race as something of equal status and not hierarchical* (Allport, 1954; Pettigrew, 1998). The intergroup contact hypothesis helps explain why people that participate in racially diverse activities or have frequent social interac-tions with other-race persons, are more likely to be in an IRR and have a racially diverse group of friends in IRRs themselves. For instance, regardless of their own racial identity, many young adults attending college tend to have racially diverse friendship networks (Stearns, Bachmann, & Bonneau, 2009), and the friendship networks of interracially dating young adults are more racially diverse than those with same-race partners (Clark-Ibanez & Femlee, 2004; Kreager, 2008; Stearns et al., 2009).

Young adults with racially diverse friendship networks also report that it is easier to date interracially because they frequently interact with members of other racial groups or have friends who date interracially themselves. This perspective is illustrated by one college student, an Asian female, that explained she and three of her close friends were all in interracial relation-ships (Clark-Ibanez & Femlee, 2004). Along these lines, a Latina college student reported it would be easy for her to date a non-Latino "because I'm involved in organizations that have people outside of my race" (p. 300). Moreover, close friends that are interracially involved are also supportive of their other friends in IRRs because the partners "make each other happy" or "they love each other and that's all that matters (Femlee, 2001: p. 1277). The sentiment of these expressions highlights how it easier for the Bridge Kids and others to engage in interracial romance when they have a racially diverse friendship network, their friends are in IRRs, and they socially interact with people from different racial backgrounds (Clark-Ibanez & Femlee, 2004; Pettigrew, 1998). This shows that people with racially diverse friendship net-works have more opportunities to form IRRs and are more apt to have friends who approve of and support interracial relationships.

Based on the tenets of the Intergroup Contact Hypothesis (Allport, 1954; Pettigrew 1998), one could argue that the views of individuals and their friends towards interracial romance is at least partially related to racial pro-pinquity. Most young adults meet their closest friends and romantic partners in their own neighborhoods or schools. Many parts of the United States are racially segregated however (Frey, 2019; Iceland & Wilkes, 2006), contribut-ing to the average American family living in moderately to highly segregated neighborhoods (Massey & Denton, 1993; Wilkes & Iceland, 2004; statisti-calatlas.com, 2018). The inverse correlation between interracial propinquity and residential segregation means people residing in segregated communities probably have fewer friends that are other-race, interracially involved, or approve of IRRs.

Comparing the racial composition of schools and census tracts data, shows the most racially segregated communities usually have the most racially segregated schools, and the most diverse communities have the most diverse schools (Billingham & Hunt, 2016; Sikkink & Emerson, 2008; Strully, 2014). As a result, youth in segregated communities have fewer opportunities for mixed-race interactions and to develop mixed-race social networks (Allport, 1954; Clark-Ibanez & Felmlee, 2004; DuBois & Hirsch, 1990). Nonetheless, greater opportunities do not necessarily translate into greater interracial romance because even when they are in racially integrated environments, not all young adults elect to engage in interracial romance. For example, Strully (2014) found that when attending racially diverse schools, Hispanic students tended to interracially date, but Black and White students still preferred to be in same-race relationships. Black females and White males were especially uninterested in interracially dating someone at their own school, which may be related to the public nature of romantic relationships and the social stigma attached to IRRs (Vaquera & Kao, 2005). Thus, some people have a number of subjective reasons for not engaging in interracial romance, even when given the opportunity in racially diverse social environments.

CONCLUSION

The beliefs and behaviors of a young adults' family and friends have a profound impact on whether they engage in interracial romance or not. On one hand, despite the growing commonality of interracial relationships, some people that are interracially involved perceive high levels of disapproval from family and friends because of their mixed-race relationship. Roughly 40 percent of Americans are still not comfortable with a family member marrying someone of another race (Wang, 2012), and about 5 percent of young adults do not believe interracial marriage is good for society (Pew Research Center, 2017). Such opposition from those closest to them, may increase the risk that the Bridge Kids and others in interracial relationships have poorer health outcomes than those in same-race relationships because of the potential double-jeopardy they face concerning the cumulative impact of increased social stressors and fewer coping resources provided by their network of family and friends.

Yet, on the other hand, countless numbers of young adults are still crossing racial lines for romance, and many believe their family and friends are supportive of their interracial relationships (Wieling, 2003; Pew Research

Center, 2017). For those young adults that do become interracially involved, there is a bi-directional relationship whereby their partner selection process and the dynamics of their relationship are greatly impacted by their family and friends, and in turn, the Bridge Kids and others in IRRs influence how their family and friends understand the concept of race, race relations, and mixed-race partnerships. Moreover, having family and friends that engage in interracial romantic relationships themselves greatly helps young adults bridge racial groups through their own interracial romance. That is to say, it is highly probable that many Bridge Kids and others in interracial relationships have happy and healthy lives thanks to their family and friends.

REFERENCES

AARP.org. (2019). *2018 Grandparents Today National Survey: General Population Report*. https://www.aarp.org/content/dam/aarp/research/surveys_statistics/life -leisure/2019/aarp-grandparenting-study.doi.10.26419-2Fres.00289.001.pdf.

Allport, G. (1954). *The nature of prejudice*. Addison-Wesley.

Bell, G. C., & Hastings, S. O. (2011). Black and White interracial couples: Managing relational disapproval through facework. Howard Journal of Communications, 22(3), 240–59.

Billingham, C. M., & Hunt, M O. (2016). School racial composition and parent choice: New evidence in preferences of white parents in the United States. *Sociology of Education, 89*(2), 99–117.

Bovier, P. A., Chamot, E., & Perneger, T. (2004). Perceived Stress, internal resources, and social support as determinants of mental health among young adults. *Quality of Life Research, 13*, 161–70.

Brooks, J. E., & Lynch, J. (2019). Partnering across race. In R. N. Roy & A. Rollins (Eds), *Biracial families: Crossing boundaries, blending cultures, and challenging racial ideologies* (pp. 61–79). Springer.

Brown, T. N., Williams, D. R., Jackson, J. S., Neighbors, H. W., Torres, M., Sellers, S. L., & Brown, K. T. (2000). Being Black and Feeling Blue: the mental health consequences of racial discrimination. *Race and Society, 2*(2), 117–31.

Browning, J. (1951). Anti-Miscegenation Laws in the United States." 1 *Duke Bar Journal, 26* 41. http://scholarship.law.duke.edu/dlj/vol1/iss1/3.

Buggs, S. G. (2019). Color, Culture, or Cousin? Multiracial Americans and Framing Boundaries in Interracial Relationships. *Journal of Marriage and Family, 81*(5), 1221–36.

Clark-Ibanez, M., & Felmlee, D. (2004). Interethnic Relationships: The Role of Social Network Diversity. *Journal of Marriage and Family, 66*(2):293–305.

Collins, W. Andrew. (2003). More than Myth: The Developmental Significance of Romantic Relationships in Adolescence. *Journal of Research on Adolescence, 13*(1), 1–24.

Connolly, J., & Goldberg, A. (1999). Romantic Relationships in Adolescence: The Role of Friends and Peers in their Emergence and Development, pp. 266–90. *The Development of Romantic Relationships in Adolescence.* Wyndol Furman, B. Bradford Brown, and Candice Feiring, editors. Cambridge University Press.

Daley, S. E., & Hammen, C. (2002). Depressive symptoms and close relationships during the transition to adulthood: Perspectives from dysphoric women, their best friends, and their romantic partners. Journal of Consulting and Clinical Psychology, 70(1), 129–41.

Doucet, F., Hall, M. R., & Giraud, M. (2019). Parenting Mixed-Race Children. In Roy, N. R., & Rollins, A. (Eds.), Biracial Families: Crossing Boundaries, Blending Cultures, and Challenging Racial Ideologies (pp. 131–58). Nature Switzerland: Springer.

Doughty, S. E., McHale, S. M., & Feinberg, M. E. (2015). Sibling experiences as predictors of romantic relationship qualities in adolescence. *Journal of Family Issues,36*(5), 589–608.

Downey, G., Bonica, C., & Rincon, C. (1999). Rejection Sensitivity and Adolescent Romantic Relationships, pp. 148–74. *The Development of Romantic Relationships in Adolescence.* Wyndol Furman, B. Bradford Brown, and Candice Feiring, editors. Cambridge University Press.

DuBois, D. l., & Hirsch, B. J. (1990). School and Neighborhood friendship Patterns of Blacks and Whites in Early Adolescence. *Child Development, 61*, 524–36.

Edmonds, C., & Killen, M. (2009). Do Adolescent's Perceptions of Parental Racial Attitudes Relate to Their Intergroup Contact and Cross-Race Relationships?. *Group Processes & Intergroup Relations, 12(1)*, 5–21.

Falci, C., & McNeely, C. (2009). Too many friends: Social Integration, Network Cohesion, and Adolescent Depressive Symptoms. *Social Forces, 87*(4), 2031–62.

Feiring, C. (1996). Concepts of romance in 15-Year-Old Adolescents. *Journal of Research on Adolescence, 6*(2), 181–200.

Femlee, D. H. (2001). No Couple Is an Island: A Social Network Perspective on Dyadic Stability. *Social Forces, 79*(4), 1259–87.

Ferraro, K., & Famer, M. (1996). Double Jeopardy to Health Hypothesis for African Americans: Analysis and Critique. *Journal of Health and Social Behavior, 37*, 27–43.

Frey, W. H. (2019). *Six maps that reveal America's expanding racial diversity.* https://www.brookings.edu/research/americas-racial-diversity-in-six-maps/.

Furman, W., & Shaffer, L. (2003). The role of romantic relationships in adolescent development, pp. 1–20. *Adolescent romantic relationships and sexual behavior: Theory, research, and practical implications.* Paul Florsheim, editor. Mahwah, NJ: Erlbaum.

Giddens A., Mitchell, D., Richard, A., & Carr, D. (Eds.). (2019). *Essentials of Sociology, 7th edition.* W. W. Norton and Company Publications.

Goffman, Erving. (1963). *Stigma.* New York: Simon & Schuster.

Gordon, M. (1964). *Assimilation in American Life: The Role of Race, Religion, and National Origin.* Oxford University Press.

Gore, S., & Aseltine Jr. R. (2003). Race and Ethnic Differences in Depressed Mood Following the Transition from High School. *Journal of Health and Social Behavior, 44*, 370–89.

Hagerman, M. A. (2017). White families and race: colour-blind and colour-conscious approaches to white racial socialization. *Ethnic and Racial Studies, 37*(14), 2598–614.

Hayslip, B., Herrington, R. S., Glover, R. J., & Pollard, S. E. (2013). Assessing attitudes toward grandparents raising their grandchildren. *Journal of Intergenerational Relationships, 11*(4), 356–79.

Hughes, D., Roriguez, J., Smith, E. P., Johnson, D. J., Stevenson, H. C., & Spicer, P. (2006). Parents' Ethnic-Racial Socialization Practices: A Review of Research and Directions for Future Study. *Developmental Psychology, 42*(5), 747–70.

Hughes, D., Witherspoon, D. P., Rivas-Drake, & West-Bey, N. D. (2009). Received ethnic-racial socialization messages and youths' academic and behavioral outcomes: Examining the mediating role of ethnic identity and self-esteem. *Cultural Diversity & Ethnic Minority Psychology, 15,* 148–60.

Hughes, D., Harding, J., Niwa, E. Y., & Toro, J. D. (2017). Racial Socialization and Racial Discrimination as Intra-and Intergroup Processes. In book: *The Wiley Handbook of Group Processes in Children and Adolescents* (pp. 241–68).

Iceland, J., & Wilkes, R. (2006). Does Socioeconomic Status Matter? Race, Class, and Residential Segregation. *Social Problems, 53*(2), 248–73.

Infoplease.com. (2020). *United States Demographic Statistics*. https://www.infoplease .com/us/census/demographic-statistics.

James, A., Coard, S.I., Fine, M., & Rudy, D. (2018). The Central Roles of Race and Racism in Reframing Family Systems Theory: A Consideration of Choice and Time. *Journal of Family Theory & Review, 10*(2), 419–33.

Jones, J. M. (2005, October 7). Most Americans Approve of Interracial Dating. *Gallup.* http://www.gallup.com/poll/19033/Most-Americans-Approve-Interracial -Dating.aspx.

Kao, G., Joyner, K., & Balistreri, K. S. (2019). *The Company We Keep: Interracial Friendships from Adolescence to Adulthood.* Russell Sage Foundation.

Kessler, R. C., Mickelson, K., & Williams, D. (1999). The Prevalence, Distribution, and Mental Health Correlates of Perceived Discrimination in the United States. *Journal of Health and Social Behavior, 40*(3), 208–30.

Killian, K. D. (2001). Reconstructing Racial Histories and Identities: The Narratives of Interracial Couples. *Journal of Marital and Family Therapy, 27*(1), 27–42.

Killoren, S., & Roach, A. L. (2014). Sibling conversations about dating and sexuality: Sisters as confidants, sources of support, and mentors. *Family Relations, 63*(2), 232–43.

Kowal, A. K., & Blinn-Pike, L. (2004). Sibling influences on adolescents' attitudes toward safe sex practices. *Family Relations, 53*(4), 377–84.

Kramer, L., Conger, K. J., Rogers, C. R., & Ravindran, N. (2019). Siblings. In B. H. Fiese, M. Celano, K. Deater-Deckard, E. N. Jouriles, & M. A. Whisman (Eds.), APA handbook of contemporary family psychology: Foundations, methods, and contemporary issues across the lifespan (pp. 521–38). American Psychological Association.

Kreager, D. (2008). Guarded Borders: Adolescent Interracial Romance and Peer Trouble at School. *Social Forces, 87*(2), 887–910.

Kuttler, A. F., & LaGreca, A. M. (2004). Linkages among adolescent girls' romantic relationships, best friendships, and peer networks. *Journal of adolescence, 27*(4), 395–414.

LaGreca, A. M., & Mackey, E. R. (2007). Adolescents' anxiety in dating situations: The potential role of friends and romantic partners. Journal of Clinical Child and Adolescent Psychology 36(4): 522–33.

LaGreca, A. M., & Lopez, N. (1998). Social anxiety among adolescents: Linkages with peer relations and friendships. Journal of Abnormal Child Psychology, 26(2), 83–94.

Laursen, Brett, and Lauri Jensen-Campbell. 1999. "The Nature and Functions of Social Exchange in Adolescent Romantic Relationships, pp. 50–74. The Development of Romantic Relationships in Adolescence. Wyndol Furman, B. Bradford Brown, and Candice Feiring, editors. Cambridge University Press.

Lee, J., & Bean, F. (2004). America's Changing Color Lines: Immigration, Race/Ethnicity, and Multiracial Identification. *Annual Review of Sociology, 30*, 221–42.

Link, S. (2009). *Socialization for Lifelong Learning.* http://www.michaelphelps.me/uploads/5/7/5/4/57542347/socialization_for_lifelong_learning_5.pdf.

McNamara, R. P., Tempenis, M., & Walton, B. (1999). *Crossing the line: interracial couples in the South.* Greenwood Publishing Group.

Massey, D. S., & Denton, N. A. (1993). *American Apartheid: Segregation and the Making of the Underclass.* Harvard University Press.

Mendelson, T., Kubzansky, L., Datta, G., & Buka, S. (2008). Relation of female gender and low socioeconomic status to internalizing symptoms among adolescents: A case of double jeopardy? *Social Science & Medicine, 66*(6), 1284–96.

Merriam-Webster Dictionary. (2022). *Friend.* https://www.merriam-webster.com/dictionary/friend.

Milevsky, A. (2011). Sibling relationships in childhood and adolescence: Predictors and outcomes. Columbia University Press.

Miller, B. (2014). What are the odds: An examination of adolescent interracial romance and risk for depression. *Youth & Society, 49*(2), 180–202.

Miller, B. (2020). Black Interracial Families in U.S. Society. In James, A. G. (Ed.), *Black Families: A Systems Approach* (pp. 88–96). Cognella Academic Press.

Miller, B., Catalina, S., Rocks, S., & Tillman, K. (2021). It Is Your Decision to Date Interracially: The Influence of Family Approval on the Likelihood of Interracial/Interethnic Dating. *Journal of Family Issues, 43*(2), 443–66.

Miller, S. C., Olson, M. A., & Fabio, R. H. (2004). Perceived Reactions to Interracial Romantic Relationships: When Race is Used as a Cue to Status. *Group Processes & Intergroup Relations, 7*(4), 354–69.

Miller, B., & Taylor, J. (2012). Racial and Socioeconomic Status Differences in Depressive Symptoms Among Black and White Youth: An Examination of the

Mediating Effects of Family Structure, Stress and Support. *Journal of Youth and Adolescence, 41*, 426–37.

Morales, E. (2012). Parental messages concerning Latino/Black interracial dating: An exploratory study among Latina/o young adults. *Latino Studies, 10*(3), 314–33.

Neblett, E. W., Smalls, C. P., Ford, K. R., Nguyen, H. X., & Sellers, R. M. (2009). Racial socialization and racial identity: African American parents' messages about race as precursors to identity. *Journal of Youth and Adolescence, 38*(2), 189–203.

Needham, B. (2008). Reciprocal relationships between symptoms of depression and parental support during the transition from adolescence to young adulthood. *Journal of Youth and Adolescence, 37*, 893–905.

Newport, F. (2013, July 25). In U.S., 87% Approve of Black-White Marriage, v. 4% in 1958. *Gallup*. http://www.gallup.com/poll/163697/approve-marriage-blacks-whites.aspx.

Okitikpi, T. (2009). *Understanding interracial relationships*. London: Russell House.

Passel, J., Wang, W., & Taylor, P. (2010, June 4). Marrying Out: One-in-Seven New U.S. Marriages is Interracial or Interethnic. *Pew Research Center's Social & Demographic Trends Project*. https://www.pewresearch.org/social-trends/2010/06/04/marrying-out/.

Pettigrew, T. F. (1998). Intergoup Contact Theory. *Annual Review of Psychology, 49*, 65–85.

Pew Research Center. (2017). *Intermarriage in the U.S. 50 Years After Loving v. Virginia*. http://www.pewsocialtrends.org/2017/05/18/intermarriage-in-the-u-s-50-years-after-loving-v-virginia/.

Prather, J. E. (1990). It's just as easy to marry a rich man as a poor one! Students'accounts of parental messages about marital partners. *Mid-American Review of Sociology, 14*(1–2), 151–62.

Prelow, H., Mosher, C., & Bowman, M. (2006). Perceived Racial Discrimination, Social Support, and Psychological Adjustment among African American College Students. *Journal of Black Psychology, 32*(4), 442–54.

Pryor, E. (2018). Love sees no color: The pervasiveness of color-blindism within black-white intimate interracial relationships. *Michigan Sociological Review, 32*, 92–130.

Rollins, A. (2019). Racial Socialization: A Developmental Perspective. In Roy, N. R., & Rollins, A. (Eds.), *Biracial Families: Crossing Boundaries, Blending Cultures, and Challenging Racial Ideologies* (pp. 159–81). Nature Switzerland: Springer.

Rong, X. L., & Fitchett, P. (2008). Socialization and Identity Transformation of Black Immigrant Youth in the United States. *Theory Into Practice, 47*(1), 35–42.

Seshadri, G., & Knudson-Martin, C. (2013). How Couples Manage Interracial and Intercultural Differences: Implications for Clinical Practice. *Journal of Marital and Family Therapy, 39*(1), 43–58.

Shih, K. Y., Chang, T. F., & Chen, S. Y. (2019). Impacts of the model minority myth on Asian American individuals and families: Social justice and critical race feminist perspectives. *Journal of Family Theory & Review, 11*(3), 412–28.

Sikkink, D., & Emerson, M. O. (2008). School choice and racial segregation in US schools: The role of parents' education. *Ethnic and Racial Studies, 31*(2), 267–93.

Solsberry, P. W. (1994). Interracial Couples in the United State of America: Implications for Mental Health Counseling. *Journal of Mental Health Counseling, 16*(3), 304–17.

Statistical Atlas. (2018). *Overview of the United States.* https://statisticalatlas.com/United-States/Overview.

Stearns, E., Bachmann, C., & Bonneau, K. (2009). Interracial Friendships in the Transition to College: Do Birds of a Feather Flock Together Once They Leave the Nest?. *Sociology of Education, 82*(April), 173–95.

Steinbugler, A. (2012). *Beyond Loving: Intimate Research in Lesbian, Gay, and Straight Interracial Relationships.* New York: Oxford University Press.

Stephens, D. P., & Fernandez, P. (2012). The Role of Skin Color on Hispanic Women's Perceptions of Attractiveness. *Hispanic Journal of Behavioral Sciences, 34*(1), 77–94.

Stocker, C. M., Burwell, R., & Briggs, M.L. (2002). Sibling conflict in middle childhood predicts children's adjustment in early adolescence. *Journal of Family Psychology, 16*(1), 50–57.

Strully, K. (2014). Racially and Ethnically Diverse Schools and Adolescent Romantic Relationships. *American Journal of Sociology, 120*(3), 750–97.

Taylor, R. J., Brown, E., Chatters, L. M., & Lincoln, K. D. (2012). Extended Family Support and Relationship Satisfaction Among Married, Cohabiting, and Romantically Involved African Americans and Black Caribbeans. *Journal of African American Studies, 16*(3), 373–89.

Thoits, P. (2011). Mechanisms Linking Social Ties and Support to Physical and Mental Health. *Journal of Health and Social Behavior, 52*(2), 145–61.

Thomas, P.A., Liu, H., & Umberson, D. (2017). Family Relationships and Well-Being. *Innovation in Aging, 1*(3), 1–11.

Tillman, K., & Miller, B. (2017). The role of family relationships in the psychological wellbeing of interracially dating adolescents. *Social Science Research, 65*, 240–52.

Tran, A. G. & Lee, R. M. (2010). Perceived Ethnic-Racial Socialization, Ethnic Identity, and Social Competence Among Asian American Late Adolescents. *Cultural Diversity and Ethnic Minority Psychology 15*(2): 169–78.

Tucker, C. J., McHale, S. M., & Crouter, A. C. (2001). Conditions of sibling support during adolescence. *Journal of Family Psychology, 15*(2), 254–71.

Van der Walt, A., & Basson, D. P. (2015). The Lived Experiences of Discrimination of White Women in Committed Interracial Relationships with Black Men. *Indo-Pacific Journal of Phenomenology, 15*(2), 1–16.

Vaquera, E., & Kao, G. (2005). Private and Public Displays of Affection Among Interracial and Intra-Racial Adolescent Couples. *Social Science Quarterly, 86*(2), 484–509.

Vasquez, J. M. (2015). Disciplined Preferences: Explaining the (Re)Production of Latino Endogamy: Table A1. *Social Problems, 62*(3), 455–75.

Wang, W. (2012, February 16). The Rise of Intermarriage: Rates, Characteristics Vary by Race and Gender. *Pew Research Center.* https://www.pewresearch.org/social-trends/2012/02/16/the-rise-of-intermarriage/.

Wang, H., Kao, G., & Joyner, K. (2006). Stability of interracial and intraracial romantic relationships among adolescents. *Social Science Research, 35*, 435–53.

White-Johnson, R. L., Ford, K., & Sellers, R. (2010). Parental racial socialization profiles: Association demographic factors, racial discrimination, childhood socialization, and racial identity. *Cultural Diversity and Ethnic Minority Psychology 16*(2), 237–47.

Whiteman, S. D., McHale, S. M., & Soli, A. (2011). Theoretical perspectives on sibling relationships. *Journal of Family Theory & Review, 3*(2), 124–39.

Wieling, E. (2003). Latino/a and White Marriages: A Pilot Study Investigating the Experiences of Interethnic Couples in the United States. *Journal of Couple & Relationship Therapy, 2*(2/3), 41–55.

Wilkes, R., & Iceland, J. (2004). Hypersegregation in the twenty-first century. *Demography, 41*, 23–36.

Williams, D. R., & Collins, C. (1995). US Socioeconomic and Racial Differences in Health: Patterns and Explanations. *Annual Review of Sociology, 21*, 349–86.

Wight, R. G., Botticello, A., & Aneshensel, C. (2006). Socioeconomic Context, Social Support, and Adolescent Mental Health: A Multilevel Investigation. *Journal of Youth and Adolescence, 35*(1), 115–26.

Woods, S. B., Priest, J. B., & Roberson, P. N. E. (2019). Family Versus Intimate Partners: Estimating Who Matters More for Health in a 20-Year Longitudinal Study. Journal of Family Psychology, 34(2), 247–56.

Yahya, S., & Boag, S. (2014). My Family Would Crucify Me!: The Perceived Influence of Social Pressure on Cross-Cultural and Interfaith Dating and Marriage. *Sexuality & Culture, 18*(4), 759–72.

Zhang, Y., & Van Hook, J. (2009). Marital dissolution among interracial couples. *Journal of Marriage and Family, 71*(1), 95–107.

Chapter 5

Building the Next Bridge

CHAPTER OVERVIEW

The Bridge Kids are those young adults who symbolize the *social bridges* connecting people separated by racial boundaries, and the distinct social experiences of many people in interracial romantic relationships (IRRs) is perhaps best understood through the lens of arguably the most influential Bridge Kids in American history, Mildred and Richard Loving. The affectionate story of Mildred and Richard Loving began in 1950 in the rural town Central Point, Virginia. Similar to other Bridge Kids who meet their partners through the social networks of their siblings, eleven-year-old Mildred Jeter met Richard Loving, the seventeen-year-old friend of her brothers Theoliver and Musiel Jeter. Like so many adolescent relationships, over time, Mildred and Richard's platonic friendship turned romantic. Despite their feelings for one another, the two young lovers had to cope with the stressors associated with a major social issue of their day, interracial romance. It was highly problematic for Mildred (who was Black–Native American) and Richard (who was White) to be interracially dating in a geographic area that was highly segregated during a time when the Virginia Racial Integrity Act of 1924 still deemed interracial relationships as illegal. Regardless of the potential criminal offense, the two grew their relationship as an eighteen-year-old Mildred became pregnant in 1958 and married twenty-four-year-old Richard in the District of Columbia later that same year.

After returning to their hometown in Virginia, Mildred and Richard had to further deal with the social stressors to which they were exposed related to being in a stigmatized relationship. This included being arrested in the dead of night for violating Virginia's anti-miscegenation laws prohibiting interracial marriage. Upon conviction of their crime, the Lovings' one-year sentence for "cohabitating as man and wife against the peace and dignity of the Commonwealth" (Levison, 2019) was suspended on the grounds they leave the state of Virginia for twenty-five years. In other words, the Lovings' sanction for being in love was to be exiled from a State with the motto that "Virginia Is for Lovers." Nevertheless, with the help of the American Civil Liberties Union (ACLU), the Lovings petitioned to have their legal conviction and social banishment from the state of Virginia overturned. In June 1967, the Supreme Court unanimously made the landmark decision to overturn the Lovings' convictions and deemed anti-miscegenation laws unconstitutional on the grounds that they violated both the due process and equal protection clauses of the 14th Amendment to the Constitution.

The prohibition of anti-miscegenation laws resulting from the *Loving vs. Virginia* case fundamentally changed U.S. society. The legalization of IRRs theoretically made the idea of race moot, as it opened the door allowing people to cross racial lines for love, romance, family formation, and procreation. It is from this perspective that this chapter focuses on the next social bridges being built by the children of the Bridge Kids, the growing Multiracial population.

MULTIRACIAL IDENTITY

The population of children born to interracial couples and who identify with two or more racial groups (*Multiracial*), are part of a new generation of Americans whose population and visibility has been increasing concurrently with the rise in interracial couples (Mather et al., 2019). In what some call the *biracial baby boom* (Cruz & Berson, 2001; Root, 1992), as the proportion of intermarriages rose from less than 1 percent of all marriages in 1970 to 10 percent in 2015 (Pew Research Center, 2017; Passel et al., 2010), Multiracial childbirths rose from 1 percent of the population to 14 percent (Livingston, 2017; Pew Research Center, 2015). In fact, the Multiracial population is currently the fastest growing racial demographic in American society as the number of adults that self-identified as Multiracial has recently grown by 500 percent from 6.8 million in 2000 to 34 million in 2020 (Humes et al., 2011; Jones et al., 2021).

In addition to being the fastest growing, the Multiracial population is also the most diverse racial demographic with at least fifty-seven different combinations (Humes et al., 2011). Despite such diversity, the vast majority of Multiracial adults (75 percent) identify as having one White and one Nonwhite parent (White-Nonwhite Multiracial) such as a White father and Asian mother, and the remaining 25 percent self-identify as having two Nonwhite (racial minority) parents (Nonwhite-Nonwhite) such as a Black father and Native American mother or a White-Asian mother and a Black-Native American father (Humes et al., 2011; Pew Research Center,

2015). Accounting for Multiracial parents is especially important to fully understand the self-identifying Multiracial population considering nearly one in four Multiracial people also have at least one Multiracial parent (Livingston, 2017). Such racial diversity among this rapidly growing population is having a profound effect on our society by blurring the color lines and people's approaches to race relations.

Racial socialization is a salient aspect of the lives of Multiracial children and their families (Rodriguez et al., 2009; Rollins, 2019). This process is especially varied for Multiracial people given their number of possible racial identities, which probably contributes to most Multiracial individuals feeling socially pressured to identify with the monoracial group they most look like or were socialized to recognize with (Poston, 1990; Pew Research Center, 2015). For example, Bratter (2007) found that children were more likely to be categorized as Multiracial when there is no racial overlap between the parents if one parent was Multiracial themselves (e.g., Asian-White Multiracial with a Black spouse, or Native-White Multiracial with a Hispanic spouse). Nonetheless, many parents still categorize their second-generation Multiracial children as monoracial which creates a *Multiracial identity gap* whereby the number of Multiracial persons significantly rises when accounting for the racial background of an individual's parents and grandparents (Pew Research Center, 2015). Hence, the true size of the Multiracial population is unknown but even larger than what the census shows.

MULTIRACIAL HEALTH

The Multiracial identity gap is just one of many issues that make investigating the health of Multiracial persons complex, and the speed at which the Multiracial population is increasing makes examining the demographics' well-being an important public health issue. Racial identity is associated with people's social experiences, stressors, coping resources, and health (Williams, 2018), however, the self and social identity of the Multiracial population is unique. Accordingly, the exceptional identity and social experiences of Multiracial persons exposes them to a variety of social stressors that likely result in health disparities among, and between, monoracial and Multiracial groups.

Miller and colleagues (2019) attempted to address this issue with their proposal of the *Racialized Experiences of Multiracial Persons* (REMP) model that examines the link between racial identity and health outcomes for the Multiracial population. The REMP hypothesizes that racial identity, SES, social experiences, and psychosocial resources significantly affect the health outcomes of Multiracial persons as well as acknowledges that phenotypic characteristics, like skin tone, influence the self-identity and social identity of Multiracial persons. The three perspectives presented in the REMP are: (1) The White Experience; (2) The Minority Experience; and (3) The Blended Race Experience.

The *White Experience* perspective refers to Multiracial persons that self-identify as either a White-Nonwhite Multiracial (e.g., White-Asian or White-Black) or monoracial White, despite having parents with different racial backgrounds. A person's choice of racial identity may be related to the fact that they look like, or are socialized to associate with being, a member of the monoracial White group (Helms, 1990; Wolfe, 2020). For example, a sample of biracial college-aged adults were asked to choose between identifying as biracial or a monoracial minority and people that identified as Asian-White were more likely to identify as biracial than Black-White or Hispanic-White persons (Townsend et al., 2012). Similarly, both Asian-White and Native American-White adults feel they have more in common with Whites than Asians or Native Americans respectively (Pew Research Center, 2015), underscoring the importance of phenotype and socialization for Multiracial identity. Furthermore, it is easier for Multiracial persons with fairer skin tones to have a *White passing* appearance that helps them evade being stigmatized as either Black or Multiracial. Accordingly, this group of White-Nonwhite Multiracials are likely to have social experiences that are similar to monoracial Whites including benefiting from white privilege and perceiving white consciousness.

The *Minority Experience* refers to Multiracial persons that identify as either White-Nonwhite (e.g., White-Black), with two Nonwhite-Nonwhite minority groups (e.g., Black-Asian or Native-Asian), or as a monoracial minority (e.g., Hispanic or Black). The racial identification of these individuals may be related to their phenotype or racial socialization factors, as skin tone plays a particularly big role in the self-identity and social identity of many Multiracials and those with brown skin have long been socially categorized as Black. For example, brown-skinned Multiracial individuals (regardless of their racial combinations) probably have experiences akin to monoracial Blacks, and since it is definitely easier to label a Multiracial person with darker skin as Black, they are probably subjected to the same forms of prejudice and discrimination experienced by monoracial Blacks (Jordan, 2014; Khanna, 2010). Similarly, Multiracial persons that identify as a monoracial minority are likely to have social experiences that reflect being a member of that particular racial group (e.g., Asian or Native American). For instance, nearly 70 percent of Black-Nonblack Multiracial adults (1) believe the world sees them as Black, as well as (2) consider their own beliefs and social experiences are similar to those of Blacks (Pew research Center, 2015).

The *Blended Race Experience* posits that people who clearly and consistently self-identify as being Multiracial have their own racial experiences that are distinct from monoracials. Such experiences may be related to family socialization (James et al., 2018) as well as the degree to which Multiracials feel connected with their family (Roy & Rollins, 2019). These individuals may also experience microaggressions and macroaggressions for identifying as Multiracial, which in turn can negatively impact their well-being (Franco and O'Brien, 2018; Miller et al., 2019). In contrast, some Multiracials may be able to engage in *identity shifting*, a unique coping resource that allows Multiracial persons to symbolically switch their racial identity according to the race of the people with whom they are interacting (Wilton, Sanchez, & Garcia, 2013).

How Multiracial persons racially identify, in terms of his or her racial composition, is strongly associated with their risk of being mentally ill. As Miller and colleagues (2019) show using nationally representative data from the National Longitudinal Adolescent to Adult Health Study (Add Health), when generally comparing people with Multiracial identities to their monoracial peers, Multiracial persons reported having worse health in terms of greater depression, lower self-esteem, lower life satisfaction, and lower self-rated health than monoracial persons. However, when separating Multiracial persons into two specific groups based on their racial identity as either White-Nonwhite (e.g., White-Hispanic, White-Native) or Nonwhite-Nonwhite (e.g., Asian-Black, Hispanic-Native), the researchers discovered that White-Nonwhite Multiracials had greater depression, lower self-esteem, lower satisfaction, and lower self-rated health, but Nonwhite-Nonwhite Multiracials had greater self-esteem and higher self-rated health than monoracial persons.

These differences indicate there are meaningful racial disparities in health among different Multiracial pairings that are related to the different racial groups with whom the person self-identifies. Specifically, Multiracial persons who only identify with racial minority groups may actually have better health than monoracial persons, but Multiracials that partially identify as White may have poorer mental and self-rated health than monoracials. In other words, Multiracials with only minority identities may have better health than both monoracials and those Multiracials with a partial White identity. This suggests that, depending on their racial identity, all Multiracials do not face an elevated risk of mental illness or generally poorer health than monoracial individuals (Shih & Sanchez, 2005). Moreover, given the number of possible Multiracial identities, there are likely significant variations in health among specific White-Nonwhite (e.g., White-Native American, White-Hispanic/Black) and Nonwhite-Nonwhite (e.g., Asian-Black, Black/Native American) pairings.

The special racial identity of Multiracial persons also plays a big role in affecting their social well-being and relationships. For instance, research from the Pew Research Center (2015) shows Black-White Multiracials report having more in common with, and feel more accepted by, Blacks than Whites. Black-Nonblack Multiracials also have closer relationships with their Black family members than their Nonblack kin. Similarly, White-Nonwhite Multiracials with no Black heritage, have closer ties to their White relatives than their Nonwhite relatives. The social well-being of Multiracial individuals therefore seems to be linked to the extent a person has Black or White heritage. Additionally, close relationships with family are associated with better mental, physical, and overall well-being (Chen & Harris, 2019; Thomas, Liu, & Umberson, 2017). However, even less is known about the physical well-being of Multiracial persons. This is an essential area of health research needed to assess if the Multiracial demographic faces greater risk of the leading causes of death in the United States, like heart disease, cancer, and diabetes (cdc.gov, 2021), and whether vulnerability to illness varies by Multiracial identity.

Beyond health outcomes, and using a stress process model perspective, painting a holistic picture of Multiracial well-being people requires more knowledge on the social stressors to which they are exposed as well as the coping resources they have available to help them mitigate their vulnerability to poor health. For instance, among Black-Hispanic people, those with darker skin tones report having poorer mental health (see Cuevas, Dawson, & Williams, 2016) than those with lighter complexions. This suggests that *colorism*, a form of prejudice or discrimination based on an individual's skin tone whereby darker skinned people are treated less favorably than those with lighter complexions (Hannon, 2015; NCCJ, 2021), appears to be one stressor that can have a significant impact on the health of Multiracial persons. Black-Hispanic Multiracials, particularly those with darker skin tones, also have an elevated risk of exposure to stressors associated with their lower SES (Costas et al., 1981; LaVeist-Ramos et al., 2012).

Multiracial persons may also experience different social stressors related to their racial identity. One is when Multiracial persons have their racial identity mislabeled. *Mislabeling* refers to "an incident where an individual describes another person's race as something different than how that person self-identifies" (McDonald et al., 2020: p. 14). Consequently, Multiracials with a racially ambiguous appearance are often identified as Black or some other racial group (Peery and Bodenhausen, 2008). Another example is that some Black-Hispanic Multiracials report experiencing microaggressions for not being "Black enough" for the Black community or not being "Hispanic enough" for the Hispanic community (Burgess, 2016). This type of *double-marginalization* (Bierly, 2020) can have a deleteriously effect a person's psychological well-being, and can easily be ubiquitously applied to those with Multiracial identities regardless of the racial combination of their background. Along these lines, Multiracials specifically report experiencing discrimination and microaggressions related to their blended racial identities from people that doubt their self-identity or view multiracial identities as abnormal, which can lead to negative attitudes, adverse self-perceptions, and other issues with emotional adjustment (Greig, 2015; Johnston & Nadal, 2010; Sanchez, 2010).

Even less is known about the coping mechanisms used by Multiracial persons to mitigate the harmful effects of social stressors and emotionally adjust to adverse social circumstances. However, using the Blended Race Experience perspective from the REMP (Miller et al., 2019) to interpret the extant research suggests some Multiracials can integrate their multiple racial identities into one fluid racial identity (Gibbs, 1998). Multiracials that embrace their blended racial backgrounds may be better able to adapt and cope with social circumstances by switching their racial identity according to the group of people with whom they are interacting (Townsend et al., 2012; Wilton, Sanchez, & Garcia, 2012). This *identity shifting* can also be used as part of one's impression management strategies for protecting the self-worth of stigmatized people (Zeigler-Hill et al., 2012). The ability to shift racial identities, in turn, may reduce or buffer Multiracial individuals from the adverse effects of stressful events related to their discriminatory experiences, which have been found to be associated with significantly lower self-rated health (Alvarez-Galvez, 2016). Thus, a more in-depth examination of the health of the Multiracial population is needed for researchers and practitioners to develop the best specialized treatments or preventative measures to help improve the lives and well-being of this diverse and rapidly growing demographic.

MULTIRACIAL PARTNER SELECTION

Because their racial identity is so diverse and complex, the Multiracial partner selection process further confounds the idea of interracial romance that separates the Bridge Kids and others in IRRs from their peers in same-race relationships (SRRs). Multiracial partnerships can, and sometimes do, completely blur the racial lines that have traditionally been used to delineate interracial couples from same-race couples. For example, how does society racially categorize couples where both partners have Multiracial identities like John Legend and Chrissy Teigen or Alicia Keys and Swizz Beats (Kasseem Dean). From this viewpoint, more so than any other racial group, the Multiracial partner selection process can profoundly impact intergroup race relations.

The issue of racially categorizing Multiracial couples is socially important because adults that self-identify as Multiracial are more likely to have interracial experiences than monoracial Blacks and monoracial Whites (Skinner & Rae, 2019). It can be argued that unless Multiracial is defined as a distinctly new racial category consisting of anyone that self-identifies with two or more racial groups, then *all* romantic relationships involving Multiracial persons are inherently interracial. This position is echoed by a Black-White Multiracial woman who stated, "I'm mixed race so no matter what relationship I have, it'll always be a mixed-race relationship" (Song, 2015: p. 105). It could therefore be disputed that two Multiracial partners, even if both identify with the same racial groups, should still be regarded as an interracial couple.

Racial identity is a particularly salient issue in the Multiracial partner selection process because their unique identity often influences the race of the partner they choose (Roberts-Clarke, Roberts, & Morokoff, 2004). For example, it is perhaps probable, but highly unprobable, that a Black-White Multiracial with one White grandparent and three Black grandparents has the same skin tone and social experiences as a Black-White Multiracial with one Black grandparent and three White grandparents. Accordingly, some Multiracial individuals with Black-White backgrounds report having difficulties dating because they are perceived as "too White" for Black people and "too Black" for White people (Henriksen & Trusty, 2004). Multiracial persons also report struggling to select a romantic partner due to fears of being rejected or culturally alienated, fear of family disapproval, or not knowing which racial groups desired them as potential partners (Gibbs & Mascowitz-Sweet, 1991; Kelcholiver & Leslie, 2007). Consequently, differences in skin tone and lived experiences, in turn, seemingly influence how Multiracial persons self-identify themselves, their partners, and their romantic relationship (Gonlin, 2020; Reece, 2019). Such challenges may reflect differences in how Multiracial persons self-identify relative to how they are socially identified by their potential partner and others.

Another influential factor in the Multiracial partner selection process is *interpersonal similarity*, which is a dimension of social distance whereby people usually have closer social ties with, and are more attracted to, those with similar characteristics as themselves (Liviatan, Trope, & Liberman, 2008; Lydon, Jamieson, & Zanna, 1988). For instance, although most Multiracial persons have monoracial partners, Multiracial people are six times more likely to have a Multiracial partner or spouse than monoracial people (Passel et al., 2010; Pew Research Center, 2015). Furthermore, Multiracials with White-Nonblack backgrounds (e.g., White-Asian or White-Native American) are perceived as being more socially similar to Whites than other racial groups. Such racialized perceptions of their identity, in turn, contribute to White-Nonblack Multiracial persons being more likely to have White partners, whereas Multiracials with White-Black backgrounds usually partner with Blacks (Qian & Lichter, 2011).

It is also important to note that, like some monoracial individuals, many Multiracial people look beyond race and select their romantic partner on the potential of being happy with that particular person (Kelcholiver & Leslie, 2007). Choosing a partner based on personally desirable characteristics rather than their race, may contribute to Multiracial people feeling more comfortable in interracial relationships than Whites and other racial minorities (Bonam & Shih, 2009). Such comfort in one's partnership may arise from Multiracial people being affiliated with multiple heritages, and therefore they are able (but not always) to at least partially identify with their partner's heritage. In other words, a Multiracial person's diverse background probably increases their ability to discover interpersonal similarities with others. Their understanding of multiple heritages may especially develop when Multiracials are socialized in a racially inclusive environment with interracially partnered parents who teach their children how to incorporate their multiple identities into one singular identity (Gibbs, 1988; Kelcholiver & Leslie, 2007). The race of one's partner may therefore be less salient in the assortative mating process of Multiracial individuals than their monoracial peers.

The potential lesser importance Multiracial person's may place on their partner's race could be related to the growing number of interracial couples with children as indicated by the thriving Multiracial population (Pew Research Center, 2015). As the number of Multiracial families continues to rise, more children are getting racially socialized from blended racial perspectives because they are being raised in households with parents belonging to different racial groups. As the primary agents of socialization, parents are instrumental in preparing their children to become socially competent members of society by teaching them the mannerisms, beliefs, and principles of the wider society (Link, 2009). Still, the growing numbers of parents who are marrying, cohabitating (Pew Research Center, 2017), and dating across racial lines serve as people worth imitating to their children by implicitly demonstrating their beliefs that interracial romance is acceptable and, perhaps for some people, preferable. Appropriately, feelings of racial acceptance and the endorsement of interracial romance are probably strongly reinforced among young adults raised in a Multiracial household by parents in an IRR. Based on their parental role models and the racial socialization an individual is likely to receive in a Multiracial family (Rollins, 2019), I would suspect that more and more parents in IRRs support their children being interracially involved as well. Parental beliefs and behaviors, in turn, may impact the attitudes and actions of the siblings, grandparents, and extended kin of the Bridge Kids and others in IRRs. In other words, more than any other racial group, young adults raised in Multiracial families may view IRRs and their families as normative.

MULTIRACIALS' FAMILIES

As more and more Multiracial individuals develop romantic partnerships and form their own families, the impact of their partner selection process will continue to extend far beyond the romantic couples themselves. Changes to the structure and interpersonal dynamics of American families are being greatly exacerbated as the rapidly growing number of IRRs clearly indicates that interpersonal race relations have shifted and the social distance between racial groups is decreasing (Allport, 1964). As a result, the Bridge Kids and other interracially involved people have increased the commonality of Multiracial families as well as precipitated an increase in the Multiracial population. Looking forward, as the growing proportion of Multiracial youth mature and become romantically involved themselves, their future families will further add to the observed demographic changes in race and race relation in the broader society. Although our knowledge at present about the families of Multiracial individuals or how Multiracial people racially identify their own second generation (plus) Multiracial children is limited (Song 2018), it is imperative to comprehend the families of Multiracial persons today, to better predict the demographics of American families in the near future.

In terms of the impact of race on their relationship, the perceptions Multiracial people have of their partner are influenced by "their own upbringing, by parents, physical appearance, and experiences of racial 'othering' and racism" (Song, 2015: p. 103). Additionally, though it seems that any romantic relationship involving a Multiracial partner would be considered an IRR (Buggs, 2019; Song, 2015), the varied perceptions of their background experiences and own racial self-identity, lead Multiracials to have dissimilar views on the types of relationship in which they are involved. However, little is known about whether Multiracial persons categorize their romantic relationship as same-race, interracial, or something more exceptional to match their own identities.

To address this issue, Song (2015) proposes there are three general explanations Multiracial persons use to categorize their romantic partnerships as either same-race or interracial relationships. The first reason is Multiracial persons that have some racial overlap with their White partner (e.g., Hispanic-White Multiracial with a White partner or Native-White Multiracial with a White partner) see themselves as the same race as their monoracial partner and view their partnership as a SRR, even if they recognize other people see them as a mixed-race couple. The second explanation is

Multiracial individuals that may have some racial overlap with their partner but still self-identify as either Multiracial or as a member of a monoracial group that differs from their partners' (e.g., Asian-White Multiracial who identifies as Multiracial with a White partner or Black-Native Multiracial who identifies as monoracial Black with a Hispanic partner), recognize their social experiences are clearly different than their partner and see themselves being in an IRR. The third explanation is that some Multiracials identify with two or more minority groups and more readily identify with the shared minority background that overlaps with the race of their minority partner (e.g., Hispanic-Native Multiracial with a Native partner or Black-Asian Multiracial with a Black partner), but still view their relationship as interracial.

Song's (2015) explanation reveals that for Multiracial persons, interpersonal similarity in terms of shared racial backgrounds between the two partners, plays a pivotal role in whether Multiracials categorize their partnerships as same-race or interracial. More specifically, Multiracial persons tend to consider their romantic relationship as IRR unless they partially identify as White *and* have a White partner. It is also worth noting Song's (2015) three explanations of relationship classification strongly align with the notions for Multiracial social experiences outlined by the Racialized Experiences of Multiracial Persons model proposed by Miller and colleagues (2019). Combined, the perspectives of Song (2015) as well as Miller and colleagues (2019) highlight the importance of how differences in racial identity and social experiences differentially impact the assortative mating and social experiences of Multiracial persons.

Having a partner from a different racial group, however, impacts the social circumstances of people in interracial relationships which in turn affects the parenting and racialization of their children. Regardless of their partner's race, the children born to Multiracial individuals are inherently Multiracial themselves, though they may not self-identify as such. The racially reframed family systems theory suggests that understanding the effects of race on families in a diverse society is important and requires some knowledge of the underlying processes families use for socializing their children to navigate a racially stratified society (James et al., 2018). For Multiracial and other parents that identify with a racial minority group, racial socialization may include conveying messages about; race, intergroup relations, racial pride, discrimination, downplaying the importance of race, and perhaps avoiding the topic (Hagerman, 2017; Hughes et al., 2017; White-Johnson, Ford, & Sellers, 2010). Additionally, because of their own backgrounds and experiences, however, Multiracial parents are able to directly relate to their Multiracial children and help them develop a healthy identity in ways monoracial parents cannot (Doucet, Hall, & Giraud, 2019).

CONCLUSION

The unique racial identity of the Multiracial population is, and will continue to, change the way current and future generations define race and classify racial groups. Some people contend that the growing prevalence of IRRs and Multiracial romance will lead to an eventual "dilution" of the concept of race whereby race will be viewed very differently by future generations (Song & Gutierrez, 2015). As a social construct, the idea of race can be diluted or deleted with little to no social impact because people's culture will remain. Through the growing Multiracial population and their effect on race relations, more people can learn more about the social traditions and cultural heritage that both distinguish, and unify, groups in a diverse society like the United States. Thus, their Multiracial children are the ultimate legacy of the Bridge Kids as they evoke social change through their ability to deconstruct conventional ideas of race, engage in interracial romance themselves, and transform the future of race relations.

As previously stated, racial identity and race relations have always been contentious issues in the United States, and they are just as important today as they were sixty or even 160 years ago. Given that the number and proportion of people engaging in IRRs are currently at an all-time high and rising while race relations are regressing (Pew Research Center, 2019), I argue examining the direct and indirect association between interracial romance and race relations is clearly one of the most salient social issues of our time. These two issues continue to shape political policies and the racial attitudes of future generations of Americans. The beliefs and behaviors of the Bridge Kids suggests many young adults *do not* want to live in a society driven by race and race-based issues. Comprehending the multitude and complexity of factors associated with interracial romance is much more than about romance, it is about understanding race relations and assimilation in a multicultural society. Ideally, our society will ultimately get to a place where race no longer matters, and we will simply refer to interracial relationships as just "relationships." When, *not if*, we get to that point, we will owe an immense thank you to the *Bridge Kids*. As such, examining the lives and well-being of the Bridge Kids and others in interracial romantic relationships is an essential part of gauging measures of health and social progression in our society.

REFERENCES

Allport, G.W. 1954. *The Nature of Prejudice*. Reading, MA: Addison-Wesley.

Alvarez-Galvez, J. (2016). Measuring the effect of ethnic and non-ethnic discrimination on European's self-rated health. *International Journal of Public Health, 61*(3), 367–74.

Bierly, R. (2020). *Afro-Latino Identities in the U.S. and Double Marginalization.* https://www.panoramas.pitt.edu/art-and-culture/afro-latino-identities-us-and-double-marginalization.

Bonam, C. M., & Shih, M. (2009). Exploring Multiracial Individuals' Comfort with Intimate Interracial Relationships. *Journal of Social Issues, 65*(1), 87–103.

Bratter, J. (2007). Will "Multiracial Survive the Next Generation?: The Racial Classification of Children of Multiracial Parents. *Social Forces, 85*(2), 821–49.

Buggs, S. G. (2019). Color, Culture, or Cousin? Multiracial Americans and Framing Boundaries in Interracial Relationships. *Journal of Marriage and Family, 81*(5), 1221–36.

Burgess, C. (2017). Having to say everyday . . . I'm not black enough . . . I'm not white enough. Discourse of Aboriginality in the Australian education context. *Race Ethnicity and Education, 20*(6), 737–51.

Center for Disease Control and Prevention. (2021, April 9). *Deaths and Mortality.* https://www.cdc.gov/nchs/fastats/deaths.htm.

Chen, P., & Harris, K. M. (2019). Association of Positive Family Relationships with Mental Health Trajectories from Adolescence to Midlife. *JAMA Pediatric, 173*(12), 1–11.

Costas, Jr. R., Garcia-Palmieri, M., Sorlie, P., & Hertzmark, E. (1981). Coronary Heart Disease Risk Factors in Men with Light Skin and Dark Skin in Puerto Rico. *American Journal of Public Health, 71*, 614–19.

Cruz, B., & Berson, M. (2001). The American Melting Pot? Miscegenation Laws in the United States. *Organization of American Historians, 15*(4), 80–84.

Cuevas, A. G., Dawson, B. A., & Williams D. R. (2016). Race and Skin Color in Latino Health: An Analytic Review. *American Journal of Public Health, 106*(12), 2131–36.

Doucet, F., Hall, M. R., & Giraud, M. (2019). Parenting Mixed-Race Children. In Roy, N. R., & Rollins, A. (Eds.), *Biracial Families: Crossing Boundaries, Blending Cultures, and Challenging Racial Ideologies* (pp. 131–58). Nature Switzerland: Springer.

Franco, M. G., & O'Brien, K. M. (2018). Racial identity invalidation with multiracial individuals: An instrument development study. *Cultural Diversity and Ethnic Minority Psychology, 24*(1), 112–25

Gibbs, J. T. (1998). Identity and Marginality: Issues in the Treatment of Biracial Adolescents. *American Journal of Orthopsychiatry, 57*(2), 265–78.

Gibbs, J. T., & Moskowitz-Sweet, G. (1991). Clinical and Cultural Issues in the Treatment of Biracial and Bicultural Adolescents. *Families in Society: The Journal of Contemporary Social Services, 72*(10), 579–92.

Gonlin, V. (2020). Colorful Reflections: Skin Tone, Reflected Race, and Perceived Discrimination among Blacks, Latinxs, and Whites. *Race and Social Problems, 12*, 246–64.

Greig, A. (2015). Understanding the Stressors and Types of Discrimination That Can Affect multiracial Individuals: Things to Address and Avoid in Psychotherapy Practice. *Psychotherapy Bulletin* 50(2): 56–60.

Hagerman, M. A. (2017). White families and race: colour-blind and colour-conscious approaches to white racial socialization. *Ethnic and Racial Studies, 37*(14), 2598–614.

Hannon, Lance. 2015. White Colorism. Social Currents 2(1): 12–21.

Helms, J. E. (Ed.). (1990). Black and White racial identity: Theory, research, and practice. Greenwood Press.

Henriksen, R. C., Jr., & Trusty, J. (2004). Understanding and Assisting Black/White Biracial Women in Their Identity Development. Women & Therapy, 27(1–2), 65–83.

Hughes, D., Harding, J., Niwa, E. Y., & Toro, J. D. (2017). Racial Socialization and Racial Discrimination as Intra-and Intergroup Processes. In book: *The Wiley Handbook of Group Processes in Children and Adolescents* (pp. 241–68).

Humes, K., Jones, N., & Ramirez, R. (2011). *Overview of Race and Hispanic Origin: 2010. U.S. Census Bureau.* http://www.census.gov/prod/cen2010/briefs/c2010br -02.pdf.

James, A., Coard, S.I., Fine, M., & Rudy, D. (2018). The Central Roles of Race and Racism in Reframing Family Systems Theory: A Consideration of Choice and Time. *Journal of Family Theory & Review, 10*(2), 419–33.

Johnston, M. P., & Nadal, K. L. (2010). Multiracial Microaggressions: Exposing Monoracism in Everyday Life and Clinical Practice. In D. W. Sue (Ed), *Microaggressions and marginality: Manifestation, dynamics, and impact* (pp. 123–44). New York: Wiley & Sons.

Jones, N., Marks, R., Ramirez, R., Rios-Vargas, M. (2021). 2020 Census Illuminates Racial and Ethnic Composition of the Country. *United States Census Bureau.* https://www.census.gov/library/stories/2021/08/improved-race-ethnicity-measures -reveal-united-states-population-much-more-multiracial.html.

Jordan, W. D. (2014). Historical Origins of the One-Drop Racial Rule in the United States. *Journal of Critical Mixed Race Studies, 1*(1): 98–132.

Kelcholiver, K., & Leslie, L. A. (2007). Biracial Females' Reflections on Racial Identity Development in Adolescence. *Journal of Feminist Family Therapy, 18*(4), 53–75.

Khanna, N. (2010). "If You're Half Black, You're Just Black": Reflected Appraisals and the Persistence of the One-Drop Rule. *The Sociological Quarterly, 51*(1), 96–121.

LaVeist-Ramos, T. A., Galarraga, J. Thorpe Jr., R.J., Bell, C. N., & Austin, C. J. (2012). Are Black Hispanics black or Hispanic? Exploring disparities at the intersection of race and ethnicity. *Journal of Epidemiology of Community Health, 16*, e21.

Levinson, S. (2019, June 12). Looking Back on Loving v. Virginia 52 Years Later. *ACLU* Virginia. https://acluva.org/en/news/looking-back-loving-v-virginia-52 -years-later.

Link, S. (2009). *Socialization for Lifelong Learning.* http://www.michaelphelps.me/uploads/5/7/5/4/57542347/socialization_for_lifelong_learning_5.pdf.

Liviatan, I., Trope, Y., & Liberman, N. (2008). Interpersonal Similarity as a Social Distance Dimension: Implications for Perceptions of Others' Actions. *Journal of Experimental Social Psychology, 44*(5), 1256–69.

Livingston, G. (2017, June 6). The rise of Multiracial and multiethnic babies in the U.S. *Pew Research Center.* https://www.pewresearch.org/fact-tank/2017/06/06/the-rise-of-Multiracial-and-multiethnic-babies-in-the-u-s/.

Lydon, J. E., Jamieson, D. W., & Zanna, M. P. (1988). Interpersonal similarity and the social and intellectual dimensions of first impressions. Social Cognition, 6(4), 269–86.

Mather, M., Jacobsen, L.A., Jarosz, B., Kilduff, L., Lee, A., Pollard, K.M., Scommegna, P., & Vanorman, A. (2019). "America's Changing Population: What to Expect in the 2020 Census," Population Bulletin 74, no. 1. https://www.prb.org/wp-content/uploads/2020/10/2019-74-1-Pop-Bulletin-Census.pdf.

McDonald, C. P., Chang, C. Y., O'Hara, C., Guvensel, K., & Parker, L. (2020). Racial Mislabeling in Multiracial Individuals: Implications for Professional Counseling and Education. *Teaching and Supervision in Counseling, 2*(1), 13–23.

Miller, B., Rocks, S., Catalina, S., Zemaitis, N., Daniels, K., & Londono, J. (2019). The Missing Link in Contemporary Health Disparities Research: A Profile of the Mental and Self-Rated Health of Multiracial Young Adults. *Health Sociology Review, 28*(2), 209–27.

NCCJ. (2021). *Colorism.* Retrieved May 1, 2020 (https://www.nccj.org/colorism-0).

Passel, J., Wang, W., & Taylor, P. (2010, June 4). Marrying Out: One-in-Seven New U.S. Marriages is Interracial or Interethnic. *Pew Research Center's Social & Demographic Trends Project.* https://www.pewresearch.org/social-trends/2010/06/04/marrying-out/.

Peery, D., & Bodenhausen, G. V. (2008). Black + White = Black: Hypodescent in Reflexive Categorization of Racially Ambiguous Faces. *Psychological Science 19*(10: 973–77.

Pew Research Center. (2015). *Multiracial in America: Proud, Diverse and Growing in Numbers.* https://www.pewresearch.org/social-trends/2015/06/11/multiracial-in-america/.

Pew Research Center. (2017). *Intermarriage in the U.S. 50 Years After Loving v. Virginia.* http://www.pewsocialtrends.org/2017/05/18/intermarriage-in-the-u-s-50-years-after-loving-v-virginia/.

Pew Research Center. (2019). *Race in America 2019.* https://www.pewresearch.org/social-trends/2019/04/09/race-in-america-2019/.

Poston, W.S.C. (1990). The Biracial Identity Development Model: A Needed Addition. *Journal of Counseling & Development, 69*, 152–55.

Qian, Z., & Lichter, D. T. (2011). Changing patterns of interracial marriage in a multiracial society. Journal of Marriage and Family, 73(5), 1065–84.

Rodriguez, J., Umana-Taylor, A., Smith, E.P., & Johnson, D.J. (2009). Cultural Processes in Parenting and Youth Outcomes: Examining a Model of Racial-Ethnic

Socialization and Identity in Diverse Populations. *Cultural Diversity and Ethnic Minority Psychology, 15*(2), 106–11.

Reece, R. L. (2019). Coloring Racial Fluidity: How Skin Tone Shaoes Multiracial Adolescents' Racial Identity Changes. *Race and Social Problems, 11*, 290–98.

Roberts-Clarke, I., Roberts, A. C., & Morokoff, P. (2004). Dating Practices, Racial Identity, and Psychotherapeutic Needs of Biracial Women. *Women & Therapy, 27*(1–2), 103–17.

Rollins, A. (2019). Racial Socialization: A Developmental Perspective. In Roy, N. R., & Rollins, A. (Eds.), *Biracial Families: Crossing Boundaries, Blending Cultures, and Challenging Racial Ideologies* (pp. 159–81). Nature Switzerland: Springer.

Root, M. P. P. (Ed.). (1992). *Racially mixed people in America.* Sage Publications, Inc.

Sanchez, D. T. (2010). How Do Forced-Choice Dilemmas Affect Multiracial People? The Role of Identity Autonomy and Public Regard in Depressive Symptoms. *Journal of Applied Social Psychology, 40*(7), 1657–77.

Shih, M. & Sanchez, D.T. (2005). Perspectives and Research on the Positive and Negative Implications of Having Multiple Racial Identities. *Psychological Bulletin, 131*(4), 569–91.

Skinner, A. L., & Rae, J, R. (2019). A Robust Bias Against Interracial Couples Among White and Black Respondents, Relative to Multiracial Respondents. *Social Psychological and Personality Science, 10*(6), 823–31.

Song, M. (2015). What Constitutes Intermarriage for Multiracial People in Britain?. *ANNALS of the American Academy of Political and Social Science, 662(*1), 94–111.

Song, M. (2018). Learning From Your Children: Multiracial Parents' Identifications and Reflections of Their Own Racial Socialization. *Emerging Adulthood, 7*(2), 119–27.

Song, M., & Gutierrez, C. O. (2015). 'Keeping the story alive': is ethnic and racial dilution inevitable for multiracial people and their children?. *The Sociological Review, 63*, 680–98.

Thomas, P.A., Liu, H., & Umberson, D. (2017). Family Relationships and Well-Being. *Innovation in Aging, 1*(3), 1–11.

Townsend, S. S., M., Fryberg, S. A., Wilkins, C. L., & Markus, H. R. (2012). Being Mixed: Who Claims a Biracial Identity?. *Cultural Diversity and Ethnic Minority Psychology, 18*(1), 91–6.

White-Johnson, R. L., Ford, K., & Sellers, R. (2010). Parental racial socialization profiles: Association demographic factors, racial discrimination, childhood social-ization, and racial identity. *Cultural Diversity and Ethnic Minority Psychology, 16*(2), 237–47.

Williams, D. R. (2018). Stress and the Mental Health of Populations of Color: Advancing Our Understanding of Race-Related Stressors. *Journal of Health and Social Behavior, 59*(4), 466–85.

Wilton, L. S., Sanchez, D. T., & Garcia, J. A. (2013). The Stigma of Privilege: Racial Identity and Stigma Consciousness Among Biracial Individuals." *Race and Social Problems, 5*(1), 41–56.

Wolfe, B. (2020, February 25). Racial Integrity Laws (1924–1930). *Encyclopedia Virginia.* https://www.encyclopediavirginia.org/Racial_Integrity_Laws_of_the_1920s.

Zeigler-Hill, V., Wallace, M. T., & Myers, E. M. (2012). Racial differences in self-esteem revisited: The role of impression management in the black self-esteem advantage. *Personality and Individual Differences, 53*, 785–89.

Conclusion

Sara Rocks and Kathryn Harker Tillman

Today's youth are coming of age during a time of tremendous racial transformation. Adolescents and young adults in the United States are increasingly likely to socialize, date, cohabit, and marry across racial/ethnic lines (Allen, 2017; Miller, 2014; Tillman & Miller 2017; Wang et al., 2006). They also are more likely than previous generations to self-identify as multiracial and to bear children with partners of a differing race/ethnicity (Joyner & Kao, 2005; Parker et al., 2015). Through interracial romantic relationships (IRRs), young people are able to form close cross-race linkages and build racially diverse social networks of family, friends, and acquaintances. As such, these "Bridge Kids" play a central role in the process through which our society is deconstructing its notions of race and reorganizing its system of race relations. These societal changes have important implications for the identities, health, and well-being of both current and future generations.

Many people, within both academia and the general public, are encouraged by these trends, viewing them as a sign that racial hierarchies and barriers are breaking down and that our society is growing increasingly inclusive (Joyner & Kao, 2005; Kennedy, 2003; Miller, 2014). Some scholars have suggested, however, that racial hierarchies and barriers are not likely to disappear. Instead, they believe we will see changes in how different groups of people are categorized and how the categories are arranged within an altered racial hierarchy (Bonilla-Silva, 2004; Ho et al., 2011; Miller et al., 2019). In particular, they question the extent to which the color line separating Black Americans from all others is moving (Lee & Bean, 2010; 2012; Sears & Savalei, 2006; Kroeger & Williams, 2011), and exactly how individuals with multiracial backgrounds will self-identify and be categorized by others (Abascal, 2020; Bonilla-Silva, 2004; Miller et al., 2019). Notions of race and ideas about appropriate interracial interactions are shifting, but not all racial/ethnic groups may experience these shifts in a similar way or at a similar pace.

The focus of this final discussion chapter is to examine some of the larger social forces that will help to shape future trends in interracial intimacy. In particular, we focus on: (1) the importance of widespread social practices and institutionalized policies that can either encourage or discourage cross-racial interactions, (2) the importance of technology and contemporary media for providing access to diverse communities, role-modeling interracial interactions, and shaping views of different racial/ethnic groups, and (3) the rise of the multiracial population and how it will likely influence racial self-identification and broader notions of race and ethnicity. We then discuss what future trends in interracial intimacy might mean for the health and well-being of the Bridge Kids' generation.

THE IMPORTANCE OF SOCIAL
PRACTICES AND POLICIES

Throughout the history of the United States, social practices and legal policies have created and perpetuated physical and social separation between people of different racial/ethnic groups. These practices and policies have shifted and changed a great deal over time, but they continue to have lasting effects on the interpersonal relationships and family formation behaviors of the current generation of young adults. After all, it has been less than sixty years since the Civil Rights Act of 1964 outlawed discriminatory practices in public accommodations and employment, the 1965 Voting Rights Act prohibited racial discrimination in voting, the 1965 Immigration Act opened up immigration to the United States from non-European nations, the 1967 Supreme Court case *Loving v. Virginia* ruled that anti-miscegenation laws were unconstitutional, and the 1968 Fair Housing Act prohibited racial discrimination in the sale or rental of real estate. We also have only recently begun to break down the long-standing social and legal practice of categorizing individuals by one, and only one, racial background, regardless of the racial complexity within their lineage. The 2000 Census was the first U.S. Census in which individuals were allowed to choose more than one racial category when describing themselves and their household members.

Although changing oppressive laws and policies is a crucial step in engendering social change, doing so does not immediately affect individuals' attitudes, preferences, and behavior, particularly in life domains that are considered private or family-related (Brinkman & Brinkman, 2005). For many young adults in the United States today, the pivotal changes in law brought about by the civil rights movement, and the well-documented social upheaval that occurred as a result of them, took place during the formative years of their grandparents' lives. Grandparents, even when not residing with their grandchildren, tend to influence attitudes and behaviors, both directly through one-on-one interactions and indirectly through their influence over the middle generation (i.e., the young people's parents) (Denham & Smith, 1989; O'Neil, 2007'; Roberto & Stroes, 1992). Given this process of inter-generational transmission, it is not surprising that social norms and practices that promote a system of racial homogamy and that discourage the formation of IRRs and multiracial families are still common. A substantial portion of adults, particularly older adults, continue to disapprove of IRRs and would be unhappy should a family member choose to marry across racial/ethnic lines (Passel et al., 2010).

In addition, the average American family continues to live and raise children in a highly segregated environment (Intrator et al., 2017; Massey, 2020), where the opportunity to meet and form intimate relationships with people of different racial/ethnic backgrounds is limited. Research also has shown that residential and social segregation of Whites tends to shape their racial attitudes and beliefs, including ideas about interracial marriage, in negative ways (Bonilla-Silva & Embrick, 2007). Contemporary segregation results from personal choices, particularly on the part of White Americans (Kye, 2018), continuing discrimination in housing and employment (Korver-Glenn, 2018; Pager & Shepherd, 2008), and numerous "race-neutral" policies that have racially discriminatory implications, such as charter or "school choice programs" (Bischoff & Tach, 2020; Roda & Wells, 2013). Although housing discrimination is illegal, research shows that discrimination in the sale and rental of real estate and in mortgage-related banking practices remains widespread and enforcement of laws quite rare (Quick & Kahlenberg, 2019; An, Orlando, & Rodnyansky, 2019). This ongoing discrimination, combined with the fact that racial/ethnic minorities have significantly lower average household income and wealth levels than do White Americans (Pew Research Center, 2016), has led to persistent racial/ethnic residential segregation and a greater concentration of poverty for communities of color (Intrator et al., 2017; Massey, 2020; Quick & Kahlenberg, 2019). At the individual level, it also means that racial/ethnic minorities, particularly Black and Latinx individuals, are less able than Whites to translate their own income or wealth into residential capital by moving into more affluent and well-resourced neighborhoods (An, Orlando, & Rodnyansky, 2019).

This residential segregation is directly linked to educational segregation, as the American public school system tends to distribute children to schools by neighborhood location and to fund schools largely through local property taxes (Ladd & Goertz, 2012). Over the past thirty years we have seen a dismantling of Civil Rights Era programs that actively sought to integrate schools by race, most notably programs that bussed students across traditional neighborhood lines, and we have watched as rates of segregation have risen to levels not seen since the 1960s (Frankenberg, Ee, & Ayscue, 2019). Even if "race-neutral" on the surface, policies that zone and fund schools by neighborhood location ensure that most children will attend schools that are highly segregated, and children of different racial/ethnic groups will attend schools that are differentially resourced. Indeed, these policies mean that even middle-class minority families, particularly Black families, have a higher likelihood of being zoned for high-poverty schools than do low-income Whites (Quick & Kahlenberg, 2019).

In recent decades, we have seen a rise in state and local policies that allow parents to engage in "school choice," through the use of charter schools, magnet schools, and lottery-based systems. While, theoretically, this should open up spots in higher funded, higher performing schools to children of all backgrounds, in practice it is more highly resourced parents who have been most able to take advantage of these programs and charter schools tend to be no less segregated than regular public schools (Bischoff & Tach, 2020; Frankenberg, Siegel-Hawley and Wang, 2011). In addition to providing different educational experiences, the effect of these educational policies is to discourage the intermingling of youth from different racial and ethnic backgrounds (Frankenberg, Siegel-Hawley & Wang, 2011; Roda & Wells, 2013), lowering their cross-group interactions and decreasing the likelihood that they will become involved in interracial friendships and romantic relationships (Clark-Ibanez & Felmlee, 2004).

Although not generally due to formal policies, religious institutions also tend to reinforce the practice of social homogamy. Most Americans continue to identify with a religious tradition and attend religious services at least sporadically (Newport, 2018), and religious institutions remain among the most highly segregated institutions in American society today (Polson & Dougherty, 2019). Often members of religious communities are encouraged by their families and peers to find romantic partners who share their same faith background (Polson & Dougherty, 2019). These social pressures tend to further limit opportunities for individuals to socialize and engage in intimate relationships with people of other racial/ethnic backgrounds, reinforcing the experiences that young people have in their neighborhoods and schools.

U.S. immigration policies and political rhetoric surrounding immigration also continue to have significant effects on interactions between individuals of different racial/ethnic groups. Even though the vast majority of immigrants in the United States are legally authorized to live and work in the country (Radford & Noe-Bustamante, 2019) and immigrants are statistically less likely to commit crimes or engage in delinquency than native-born individuals (Adelman et al., 2017; Bersani, 2014), our recent political discourse surrounding immigrants has been shaped largely by fear of terrorism, crime, and undocumented immigration (Cohn, 2015). Recent opinion polls indicate that overall perceptions of immigrants in the United States have not become more negative over the past decade (Radford & Noe-Bustamante, 2019), but popular press and media reports do suggest that the expression of anti-immigrant sentiments in public settings has become more common and more blatantly racist. In particular, we have seen a rise in public expression of hostility toward immigrants from Latin America and predominantly Muslim countries, including public statements made by President Trump and those in his administration. Over the past decade, the U.S. government also has significantly tightened immigration laws, making legal immigration more difficult and increasing deportations of long-term residents, including those who have U.S.-citizen spouses and children (Cohn, 2015; Radford & Noe-Bustamante, 2019). Most recently we also have seen attempts to reduce protections for unauthorized immigrants who were brought to the United States as children (Krogstad, 2017). Together, these forces have reduced relationship and family stability for many who are involved, or who might consider being involved, in an interracial/interethnic relationship that includes a non-citizen.

Overall, then, the evidence suggests that most young people in the United States regularly find themselves surrounded by social norms and institutionalized policies that work to keep them physically and socially apart from peers of different racial/ethnic backgrounds, even if they and their families have relatively open and progressive ideas. Researchers Quick and Kahlenberg (2019) argue that this systemic racial separation was first engineered through government policies and, therefore, will need government action to dismantle them. The "Bridge Kids" generation may be our best hope of motivating such action. As these young people age, they will begin to take positions that directly influence the policies affecting the day-to-day lives of Americans. In addition, these young people have been raised in a technology and digital media-infused world and are well-positioned to use these tools to advocate for social change, to continue the racial deconstruction process on both societal and individual levels, and to encourage interracial friendships and intimacy despite physical segregation.

The Importance of Technology and the Media

Over the course of the last half century, we have seen radical advances in the types of technologies available to average people and the rapidity with which technological innovations are diffused throughout a society. Such rapid technological change has provided access to increasingly diverse media and has substantially increased opportunities for engagement with a variety of people across vast geographical locations. These new opportunities for engagement, in turn, encourage the formation of increasingly diverse social networks.

In the not-so-distant-past, most Americans got their news from the local paper and a small number of network television channels. With the advent of cable television, streaming services, the internet, and ever-evolving social media platforms, information now can be obtained on-demand from a seemingly unlimited number of outlets, many of which cater to clientele with particular interests and ideological leanings. We also have seen an ever-expanding set of options for obtaining visual media entertainment, such as television shows, movies, and user-created content (e.g., YouTube, Instagram, and TikTok videos). These innovations have increased access to media sources that include increasingly positive representation of people of color and intimate relationships that cross racial/ethnic lines (Larson, 2002; Nilson & Turner, 2014), influencing social perceptions and challenging traditional social norms. In these ways, technology and the media may have contributed to more widespread acceptance of interracial interaction, friendship, and romance. The rise of social media, in particular, also has provided people with the practical means to be exposed to, and make social connections with, a wide array of people, many of whom do not live near them and/or they may never have met in person. As such, people who live in highly segregated areas have the ability to join racially diverse virtual communities. Because the likelihood of interracial romance appears strongly tied to the racial diversity of one's social network (Clark-Ibanez & Felmlee, 2004), people with more racially diverse networks have greater opportunities to date interracially and to have friends who would accept and support interracial relationships. Indeed, some recent research suggests that couples who first meet one another online are more likely to be interracial than are couples who first meet in person (Thomas, 2020).

On the other hand, while innovations in technology and the media may have broadened our ability to access a diverse array of news, entertainment, and social platforms, they also have allowed people to choose to selectively expose themselves only to those outlets that conform to their pre-existing ideological views of the world. This tendency has risen in tandem with a growing distrust of mainstream media outlets, corporations, and government representatives, a trend particularly pronounced among the young (Raine & Perrin, 2019). Although the Bridge Kids generation is actively developing new technological resources for education and information dissemination and we have seen increasingly frequent calls for teaching digital literacy (Leaning, 2019), the selective nature of contemporary news consumption and the rapidly increasing reliance on alternative media outlets has helped to facilitate the rise of ideologically driven and divisive "fake news" (Lazer, Baum & Yochai, 2018). Social media also has allowed for people to express negative sentiments and opinions in a much more "impersonal" or anonymous way than ever before, leading to a rise in public hate-speech and inflammatory rhetoric (Mondal, Silva & Benevenuto, 2017). The extent to which this is becoming more normalized within our society is illustrated by the fact that our current political leadership chooses to regularly use social media platforms, such as Twitter, to disperse what many consider to be overtly racialized rhetoric aimed at people of color, immigrants, and non-Christians. This rhetoric actively encourages the continuation of traditional views on race and racist stereotypes, particularly among White Americans who do not have much firsthand interaction with those who are different from themselves.

Some scholars also propose that the way our contemporary media portray people of color and issues of race has encouraged a crisis of "color-blind" racism among young White Americans (Nilson & Turner, 2014). Color-blind racism, the belief that racial discrimination is no longer a driving factor behind existing racial inequalities in the United States (Bonilla-Silva, 2003; 2015), may be heightened when TV shows and movies show overly idealized visions of multiracial friendship networks, schools, and neighborhoods and news stories highlight extraordinarily successful people of color (e.g., President Barack Obama, Oprah Winfrey, and Tiger Woods) without placing into context the relative rarity of their experiences. Despite the fact that these images stand in stark contrast to the lived experience of most Americans, they suggest to many young White people that—out there in the world—racism no longer "matters" for where one lives, with whom one interacts, or the educational and employment opportunities one faces. The explanation for racial inequality then becomes one based not on racial discrimination, but on "cultural" and behavioral differences or individual failings. The end result is a perpetuation of racial stereotypes, social distancing and a lack of will to effect systematic changes that would reduce segregation and inequality.

The extent to which this color-blind racism can be upended by media reporting during particular moments of racial injustice and unrest remains to be seen. During the summer of 2020, we began witnessing one of the largest, nationwide movements to protest racial injustice and police brutality against Black Americans that we have seen in decades. Media reports of the brutal incidents that led up to these protests, in particular the murders of George Floyd, Breonna Taylor, and Ahmaud Arbery, as well as round-the-clock coverage of the protests, police violence, looting, and rioting that are sweeping the country, are inevitably shaping Americans' perceptions of race, race relations and identity. Support for the protests and police reform is high, particularly among the young (Parker et al., 2020), and current protests are drawing racially diverse crowds of protestors who are united in their fight for racial equality and justice. At the same time, color-blind racism has impeded many Americans' ability to understand the systemic roots of the problems being protested (Bonilla-Silva, 2003; Buggs, 2017; Hagerman, 2018). Selective viewing of media outlets also means different groups of Americans are being exposed to different interpretations of events, and even different "facts" about them, potentially undermining cross-group relationships and pushing us further apart. For some White Americans, this moment appears to be leading to an increased awareness of racial inequality and a motivation to discuss race, racism, and oppression in the context of their intimate relationships. Yet, current media reports also seem to be generating distrust, fear, and uncertainty among the masses, particularly those in younger generations.

Despite the potentially countervailing effects of contemporary media, there is no question that the current generation has grown up with greater access than their elders to racially diverse media representations and role models and the kinds of technology that allow for connection with diverse social networks. As a result, there exists greater opportunities to become involved in IRRs and to experience messages of social support for interracial relationships. It is the hope of many that today's young people, and those whom we have called the "Bridge Kids" in particular, will continue to use innovations in technology and the media to break down conventional notions of race, connect people of different groups, and create new bridges of racial understanding.

THE RISE OF THE MULTIRACIAL POPULATION

In addition to the existence of interracial unions, another measurable outcome associated with interracial intimacy can be found in the births of children with multiracial backgrounds. The increase in interracial partnerships, as well as the reduction of stigma surrounding them, has coincided with a well-documented "biracial baby boom" (Cruz & Berson, 2001). Although the recorded proportion of infants who are multiracial rose from roughly 1 percent of the population in 1970 to 14 percent in 2015 (Cruz & Berson, 2001; Livingston, 2017), the true extent of the rise is somewhat difficult to ascertain. Vital statistics records that use birth certificate information suggest that the number of children born to interracial pairings has risen quite steeply (Parker & Madans, 2002), but many other commonly used sources of population data, such as the U.S. Census, have only recently allowed people to identify themselves or their children as having more than one racial background. This change in data collection method has not only allowed for the more accurate representation of racial background for those with mixed-race heritage, but it has also served to socially legitimize multiracial identities and families (Parker et al., 2015). As such, a portion of the "biracial baby boom" over the past couple of decades is very likely due to the collection of more accurate and detailed data and to shifting norms surrounding self-identification.

Prior to the year 2000, the U.S. Census and many other governmental agencies/programs required individuals to identify themselves and their children on forms using only one racial category. This practice was based on the long-standing social norms and (previously enforced) legal practices associated with the "one drop rule," a convention used to sort individuals into discrete racial categories and to label them as White only if there was no evidence of any other racial/ethnic ancestry, particularly Black ancestry (Roth, 2005; Wolfe, 2015). Allowing individuals to choose more than one category resulted from shifting ideas about race and interracial childbearing and, in turn, changed our understanding of the U.S. population. In the 2000 Census, the first year to introduce this choice, 2.4 percent of the U.S. population identified as more than one race. By 2010, this sub-population had grown by about one-third, increasing to 2.9 percent of the U.S. population. During this period of time, the number of Americans checking both the "Black" and "White" boxes on the Census forms had grown by a staggering 134 percent (Jones and Bullock 2012). While some of this dramatic rise is due to increasing numbers of births to interracial partners, the rate of increase suggests that changes in how people self-identify are also substantial and that our collective understanding of racial identity has continued to change over time. At the same time, recent research reveals that a sizeable minority of children born to mixed-race partners continue to be identified by their parents as monoracial, indicating that multiracial children remain seriously undercounted (Lichter & Qian, 2018; Parker & Madans, 2002).

Despite the widespread move to a "choose all that apply" format on forms collecting demographic information, as well as a rising movement to embrace multiracial identities, social pressure to identify as monoracial has not yet disappeared from our society. To see evidence of this, one only need look at examples of famous individuals, such as President Barack Obama, U.S. Vice President Kamala Harris, and sports legend Tiger Woods. These individuals are understood to be Black by most Americans, despite common knowledge of their multiracial backgrounds and, in the case of Tiger Woods in particular, their public attempts to identify as multiracial. While this social pressure affects all people of color, it is particularly aimed at individuals with Black ancestry (Roth, 2005). Evidence of a continuing pattern of "Black exceptionalism" that maintains greater social distance between individuals with Black ancestry and Whites (and all other groups) than is the case for other historically disadvantaged groups (Kroeger & Williams, 2011; Lee & Bean, 2010, 2012; Sears & Savalei, 2006). As a result, not only are Black Americans less likely to engage in IRRs than their Asian, Latinx, and Native American peers (Kreager, 2008; Vaquera & Kao, 2005; Wang, Kao, & Joyner, 2006), but they also are less able and/or willing to claim a multiracial identity, even when they are born to parents of different racial/ethnic backgrounds.

What do these trends mean for ideas about race and interracial relationships in our broader society? The growing recognition and social legitimation of multiracial identities inherently challenges our traditional notions of race and racial categorization. While not the only factor behind the growing numbers of self-identified multiracial individuals, IRRs that lead to family formation and/or childbearing are a big part of the story. In turn, individuals from multiracial families may play an integral role in the continuing rise in IRRs, as they are more often in the position to develop extended interracial social networks by connecting relatives and friends of differing racial backgrounds and are more likely to feel supported if they choose to cross racial boundaries for romance. Thus, in general, these trends suggest that we will see a continual movement towards the deconstruction of race as we now know it.

Some scholars argue, however, that the meaning of race will undoubtedly continue to shift, but that racial boundaries and barriers will not simply blur and disappear. Rather, they propose that social norms reinforcing "Black exceptionalism" will remain, and that our understanding of race in the U.S. will shift from one largely built upon a "White/non-White" dichotomy to one largely built on a "Black/non-Black" dichotomy (Kroeger & Williams, 2011) or to a tripartite system of "White," "Honorary White," and the "collective Black," with the latter category including all people with Black heritage (Bennett, 2011; Bonilla-Silva, 2004).

More recently, some scholars have modified Bonilla Silva's tripartite system of race to more fully encompass the experience of multiracial individuals. For example, Miller and colleagues (2019) identify three general types of social experiences faced by multiracial individuals: (1) The White Experience; (2) The Minority Experience; and (3) The Blended Race Experience. Multiracial individuals who have the "White experience" tend to be identified by others as White due to phenotypical and social characteristics, and generally self-identify as White-Nonwhite (e.g., White-Asian or White-Latinx) or monoracial White, despite having parents with at least two different racial/ethnic backgrounds. This group is most likely to have social experiences similar to monoracial Whites, including the experience of *white privilege* and *white consciousness* (Miller et al., 2019). Individuals who have the "Minority experience" tend to be identified by others as Nonwhite, particularly on the basis of skin tone and other phenotypical characteristics. They can self-identify in a variety of ways, however: as White-Nonwhite (e.g., White-Black), with two distinct racial/ethnic minority groups (e.g., Black-Asian or Native American–Asian), or as a monoracial minority (e.g., Asian or Black). This group is most likely to have social experiences similar to those of their monoracial peers from racial/ethnic minority backgrounds, even if they have a White parent.

Finally, those who appear more racially ambiguous (Abascal, 2020) or who clearly self-identify as being a member of a multiracial group with experiences that are distinct from those of monoracial individuals, whether White or minority, would be categorized under the "Blended Race Experience" (Miller et al., 2019). Individuals within this group may not be as clearly and consistently categorized by other people (Abascal, 2020) and may be able to symbolically switch their identity according to the race of the people with whom they are interacting (Wilton, Sanchez, & Garcia, 2013). Although they may experience micro- and macro-aggressions for identifying as multiracial, this *identity shifting* can allow multiracial individuals to draw on various psychosocial resources that protect their mental health or filter out emotionally detrimental social experiences associated with minority status (Alvarez-Galvez, 2016; Miller et al., 2019; Shih et al., 2019; Zeigler-Hill et al., 2012).

While scholars may debate the specific changes happening to the structure of our racial classification system, the evidence suggests that our ideas of race and racial identity are continuing to shift and that the Bridge Kids are active agents of change in that process. The extent to which current trends in IRR engagement and multiracial identification end up connecting people of different races and diminishing racial barriers for individuals of all backgrounds remains to be seen, however. Progress along these lines may be very uneven across racial/ethnic groups.

THE IMPLICATIONS FOR FUTURE
HEALTH AND WELL-BEING

Despite the continuation of social norms and policies that work to keep young Americans physically and socially apart from peers of different racial/ethnic backgrounds, we expect that trends in contemporary media and technology use, the rise of the multiracial population, and the growing acceptance of multiracial identities will lead to an even higher proportion of youth engaging in IRRs. This has important implications for the future health and well-being of our population.

As discussed in depth in Chapter 4, research shows that individuals engaging in IRRs tend to experience poorer mental health outcomes and social well-being than do those in same-race relationships (Tillman & Miller, 2017; Bratter & Eschbach, 2006; Kroeger & Williams, 2011; Miller, 2014). There also is some research suggesting that adults in IRRs experience poorer physical health outcomes (Berger & Sarnyai, 2015; Yu & Zhang, 2017). Given the expectation that IRRs will increase in prevalence over time, this could lead to fears that we will see declining health outcomes in the general population. Yet, the diminished well-being of those who cross racial boundaries in their intimate relationships appears to be, in large part, a result of heightened levels of psychological stress derived from a lack of social support (Wang, Kao & Joyner, 2006), more negative parent-child relationships (Miller, 2014; Tillman & Miller, 2017), greater exposure to negative stigmas, and more experience with racially motivated discrimination (Bratter & Eschbach, 2006; Kroeger & Williams, 2011).

Not only does heightened stress undermine mental health and strain interpersonal relationships, research shows that psychological stress also can "get under the skin" to influence hormonal regulation and physiological functioning in ways that increase the likelihood of both acute and chronic physical health conditions (Berger & Sarnyai, 2015; Turner, 2013). As IRRs become more common-place and garner more social recognition, and the meaning of racial categories continues to shift and blur, we may see fewer and fewer differences in the stress exposure of young people who form relationships with same-race and different-race partners. As a result, we also may see a reduction rather than an increase in overall mental health and well-being disparities among American youth. Given that mental and social well-being during adolescence and the early adult years is strongly associated with well-being throughout adulthood (Lewinsohn et al., 2003), any such reduction could have important enduring consequences for decades to come.

It is important to keep in mind, however, that the anticipated decrease in stress exposure may not accrue equally to people of all racial/ethnic backgrounds or within all types of IRRs. Previous studies reveal that Black individuals in IRRs and those in interracial partnerships that include one Black partner are the most likely to report increased stress as a result of family disapproval of their relationship (Bell & Hastings, 2015; Childs 2005; Miller et al., 2004; Morales, 2012); and experiences of discrimination while in public (Kroeger & Williams, 2011; Van der Walt & Basson, 2015). Coresidential couples in IRRs that include one Black partner also appear to be less able to use their income to move out of high-poverty neighborhoods than their peers, despite attempts to migrate toward more well-resourced areas (Gabriel, 2018). Finally, ongoing research suggests that partners in Black-Nonblack unions engage in substantially more race-based emotion work than do those in other types of interracial unions, and that the burden of this added labor is especially pronounced for the Black partners who already face heightened stress as a result of their individual experiences with racism and discrimination (Tillman et al., unpublished).

These findings, combined with the patterns of "Black exceptionalism" noted above, suggest that IRRs that include Black partners may continue to generate higher levels of stress that diminish health and well-being (particularly for the Black partner), even as other types of interracial pairings become less consequential for these outcomes. Given the findings to date, future research on the health outcomes of American youth must pay more attention to the interconnections between racial/ethnic self-identification, engagement in interracial unions, experience with discrimination and stigma, and indicators of mental and physical well-being. Doing so will not only help us to better understand current health trends, but it will also allow us to better predict future health outcomes in our society and promote health and well-being for all.

CONCLUSION

As the evidence throughout this text shows, today's youth are taking their place in history as a generation touched by, and integral to, fundamental changes in our society's ideas about racial categorization, racial/ethnic identity, and appropriate interactions between people of different racial and ethnic groups. The Bridge Kids, those who purposefully engage in interpersonal relationships that cross traditional racial/ethnic lines, are crucial agents of social change, confronting and deconstructing long-standing beliefs and social norms and bridging together families, friends and communities that might not otherwise interact. In doing so, they are actively transforming both their individual and collective futures.

The growing pervasiveness of IRRs among American youth can be seen as an indicator of our society's increasing willingness to allow racial assimilation and as evidence of declining racial/ethnic prejudice and discrimination (Gordon, 1964; Joyner & Kao 2005; Kennedy, 2003; Miller, 2014). While it is difficult to project exactly how the trends discussed here will influence our larger society over time, evidence suggests that the meaning of race will likely continue to shift and many of our current racial distinctions will become less salient. Overall, we anticipate that this will be beneficial to our society by reducing racial barriers and divisions and lowering the stigma and discrimination faced by those who push back against norms of racial homogamy in their relationships and families. This, in turn, will benefit the health and social well-being of a great number of current and future Americans.

The process of racial deconstruction will not likely proceed, however, at the same pace for all groups and will not necessarily lead to equality of social power within our society. For example, research uncovering patterns of "Black exceptionalism" indicate that our society may hold a future where Whites, Asians, Native Americans, and Latinx individuals increasingly intermingle, forming interracial relationships and multiracial families more readily than ever, but where Blacks continue to face heightened levels of exclusion and discrimination (Kroeger & Williams, 2011; Lee & Bean, 2010, 2012; Sears & Savalei, 2006). It is also possible that, regardless of shifting ideas about the social acceptability of IRRs and multiracial identities, monoracial Whites and those in same-race White partnerships will continue to retain significantly greater social and political power due to their greater access to socioeconomic resources. White Americans continue to have higher average incomes, experience greater employment opportunities, and receive larger intergenerational transfers of family wealth that was derived from historical practices of discrimination (Pew Research Center, 2016). Thus, we may still have a long way to go to address the ramifications of white supremacy for the structure of power within our country.

So, where will all of this lead us as a nation? We, the authors, have a lot of hope for the future of race relations in the United States, in large part because of the Bridge Kids. Although progress certainly will not occur in a straight, unbroken line, these young people are actively reshaping our society in ways that ultimately will lead to more tolerance, more inclusion, and a better quality of life for future generations of Americans. They are reaching their adult years primed to use rapidly advancing technology and media resources to break down stereotypes, develop diverse networks, and advocate for social change. Moreover, they will soon be of an age to hold leadership positions with the power to enact real, structural changes to the institutional policies that have long enforced racial and ethnic separation and impeded racial justice. For all of these reasons, we see great potential in the Bridge Kids' ability to lead this nation towards a more promising future.

REFERENCES

Abascal, M. (2020). Contraction as a Response to Group Threat: Demographic Decline and Whites' Classification of People Who Are Ambiguously White *American Sociological Review*, 85(2), 298–322.

Adelman, R., Williams, L. R., Markle, G., Weiss, S., & Jaret, C. (2017). Urban Crime Rates and the Changing Face of Immigration: Evidence across four decades. *Journal of Ethnicity in Criminal Justice*, 15(1), 52–77.

Allen, C., (2017). The Attitudes and Stigmas Surrounding Modern Day Interracial Relationships, *Siegel Institute Ethics Research Scholars*: Vol. 2, Article 3. Available online: https://digitalcommons.kennesaw.edu/siers/vol2/iss1/3. [Accessed June 16, 2020].

Alvarez-Galvez, J. (2016). Measuring the Effect of Ethnic and Non-Ethnic Discrimination on Europeans' Self-Rated Health. *International Journal of Public Health*, 61(3), 367–74.

An, B., Orlando, A., & Rodnyansky, S. (2019). The Physical Legacy of Racism: How Redlining Cemented the Modern Built Environment" *SSRN Electronic Journal.* Available online: https://ssrn.com/abstract=3500612. [Accessed June 16, 2020].

Bell, G. C., & Hastings, S. O. (2015). Exploring Parental Approval and Disapproval for Black and White Interracial Couples. *Journal of Social Issues, 71*(4), 755–71

Bennett, P. R. (2011). The Social Position of Multiracial Groups in the United States: Evidence from Residential Segregation, *Ethnic and Racial Studies*, 34(4), 707–29.

Berger, M. M., & Sarnyai, Z. (2015). More Than Skin Deep: Stress Neurobiology and Mental Health Consequences of Racial Discrimination *Stress,* 18(1), 1–10.

Bersani, B. E. (2014). Examination of First- and Second-Generation Immigrant Offending Trajectories. *Justice Quarterly*, 31(2), 315–43.

Bischoff, K., & Tach, L. (2020). School Choice, Neighborhood Change, and Racial Imbalance Between Public Elementary Schools and Surrounding Neighborhoods. *Sociological Science*, 7, 75–99.

Bonilla-Silva, E. (2003). *Racism without Racists: Color-Blind Racism and the Persistence of Racial Inequality in the United States*. Lanham, MD: Rowman and Littlefield.

Bonilla-Silva, E. (2004). From Bi-racial to Tri-racial: Towards a New System of Racial Stratification in the USA. *Ethnic and Racial Studies,* 27(6), 931–50.8

Bonilla-Silva, E. (2015). The Structure of Racism in Color-Blind, "Post-Racial" America. *American Behavioral Scientist*, 59(11), 1358–76.

Bonilla-Silva, E., & David, E. G. (2007). "Every Place has a Ghetto . . . ": The Significance of Whites' Social and Residential Segregation. Symbolic Interaction, 30(30), 323–45.

Bratter, J., & Eschbach, K. (2006). What about the couple? Interracial marriage and psychological distress. *Social Science Research*, 35, 1025–47.

Brinkman, R. L., & Brinkman, J. E. (2005). Cultural Lag: A Relevant Framework for Social Justice. International *Journal of Social Economics*, 32(3), 228–48.

Buggs, S. G. (2017). Dating in The Time of #Blacklivesmatter: Exploring Mixed-Race Women's Discourses of Race and Racism. *Sociology of Race and Ethnicity*, 3(4), 538–51.

Childs, E. C. (2005). *Navigating Interracial Borders: Black-White Couples and Their Social Worlds.* New Brunswick, NJ: Rutgers University Press.

Clark-Ibanez, M., & Felmlee, D. (2004). Interethnic Relationships: The Role of Social Network Diversity. Journal of Marriage and Family, 66(2):293–305.

Cohn, D. (2015). How U.S. Immigration Laws and Rules Have Changed Through History. *Pew Research Center*. Available online: https://www.pewresearch.org/fact-tank/2015/09/30/how-u-s-immigration-laws-and-rules-have-changed-through-history/. [Accessed June 15, 2020].

Cruz, B. C., & Berson, M. J. (2001). The American Melting Pot? Miscegenation Laws in The United States. *OAH Magazine of History,* 15(4), 80–84.

Denham, T. E., & Smith, C. W. (1989). The influence of grandparents on grandchildren: A review of the literature and resources. *Family Relations, 38*, 345–50.

Frankenberg, E., Jongyeon, E., Ayscue, J.B., & Orfield, G. (2019). Harming our Common Future: America's Segregated Schools 65 Years after Brown. *The Civil Rights Project.* Center for Education and Civil Rights. Available online: https://www.civilrightsproject.ucla.edu/research/k-12-education/integration-and-diversity

/harming-our-common-future-americas-segregated-schools-65-years-after-brown/ Brown-65-050919v4-final.pdf. [Accessed June 14, 2020].

Frankenberg, E., Siegel-Hawley, G., & Wang, J. (2011). Choice Without Equity: Charter School Segregation. *Education Policy Analysis Archives*, 19, 1–96.

Gabriel, R. (2018). Gender and the Residential Mobility and Neighborhood Attainment of Black-White Couples. *Demography*, 55, 459–84.

Gordon, M. (1964). *Assimilation in American Life: The Role of Race, Religion, and National Origin*. New York: Oxford University Press.

Hagerman, M. (2018). *White Kids: Growing Up with Privilege in a Racially Divided America*. New York: NYU Press.

Ho, A. K., Sidanius, J., Levin, D. T., & Banaji, M. R. (2011). Evidence for Hypodescent and Racial Hierarchy in the Categorization and Perception of Biracial Individuals. *Journal of Personality and Social Psychology*, 100(3), 492–506.

Intrator, J., Tannen, J., & Massey, D. S. (2017). Segregation by Race and Income in the United States 1970–2010. *Social Science Research*, 60, 45–60.

Jones, N., & Bullock, J. (2012). The Two or More Races Population: 2010. *2010 Census Briefs*. U.S. Census. Available online: https://www.census.gov/prod/ cen2010/briefs/c2010br-13.pdf [Accessed July 20, 2020].

Joyner, K., & Kao, G. (2005). Interracial Relationships and the Transition to Adulthood. *American Sociological Review* 70(4):563–81.

Kennedy, R. (2003). *Interracial Intimacies Sex, Marriage, Identity, and Adoption*. Pantheon.

Korver-Glenn, E. (2018). "Compounding Inequalities: How racial stereotypes and discrimination accumulate across the stages of housing exchange." *American Sociological Review*, 83(4), 627–56.

Kreager, D. (2008). Guarded Borders: Adolescent Interracial Romance and Peer Trouble at School. *Social Forces* 87(2), 887–910.

Kroeger, R., & Williams, K. (2011). Consequences of Black Exceptionalism? Interracial Unions with Blacks, Depressive Symptoms, and Relationship Satisfaction. *The Sociological Quarterly*, 52, 400–20.

Krogstad, J. M. (2017). DACA has shielded nearly 790,000 young unauthorized immigrants from deportation *Pew Research Center, FactTank*. Available online: https:// www.pewresearch.org/fact-tank/2017/09/01/unauthorized-immigrants-covered-by -daca-face-uncertain-future/. [Accessed June 16, 2020].

Kye, S. H. (2018). The Persistence of White Flight in Middle-Class Suburbia. *Social Science Research*, 72, 38–52.

Ladd, H. F., & Goertz, M. E. (2012). *Handbook of Research In Education Finance And Policy*. Routledge.

Larson, M. S. (2002). Race and Interracial Relationships In Children's Television Commercials. *Howard Journal of Communications*, 13:3, 223–35.

Lazer, D. M., *et al.*(2018). The Science of Fake News. SCIENCE, March 9, 1094–96.

Leaning, M. (2019). An Approach to Digital Literacy through the Integration of Media and Information Literacy. *Media and Communication*, 7(2), 4–13.

Lee, J., & Bean, F. D. (2010). *The Diversity Paradox: Immigration and the Color Line in 21st Century America*. New York: Russell Sage Foundation.

Lee, J., & Bean, F. D. (2012). A Postracial Society or A Diversity Paradox? Du Bois Review: Social Science Research on Race, 9(2), 419–37. Bulletin, 32, 40–51.

Lewinsohn, P. M., Rohde, P., Seeley, J. R., Klein, D. N., & Gotlib, I. H. (2003). Psychosocial Functioning of Young Adults Who Have Experienced and Recovered from Major Depressive Disorder During Adolescence. Journal of Abnormal Psychology, 112(3), 353–63.

Lichter, D. T., & Qian, Z. (2018). Boundary Blurring? Racial Identification among the Children of Interracial Couples, Annals *of the American Academy of Political and Social Science*, 677(1), 81–94.

Livingston, G., & Brown, A. (2017). Intermarriage in the U.S. 50 Years after Loving v. Virginia. *Pew Research Center*. Retrieved October 1, 2021. (https:// www.pewresearch.org/social-trends/2017/05/18/intermarriage-in-the-u-s-50-years -after-loving-v-virginia/) [Accessed June 16, 2020].

Massey, D. (2020). Still the Linchpin: Segregation and stratification in the USA. *Race and Social Problems*, 12(1), 1–12.

Miller, B. (2014). What are the Odds: An Examination of Adolescent Interracial Romance and Risk for Depression. *Youth & Society*, 49(2), 180–202.

Miller, B., Rocks, S., Catalina, S., Zemaitis, N., Daniels, K., & Londono, J. (2019). The Missing Link in Contemporary Health Disparities Research: A Profile of the Mental and Self-Rated Health of Multiracial Young Adults. *Health Sociology Review, 28*(2), 209–27.

Miller, S. C., Olson, M. A., & Fabio, R. H. (2004). Perceived Reactions to Interracial Romantic Relationships: When Race is Used as a Cue to Status. *Group Processes & Intergroup Relations, 7*(4), 354–69.

Mondal, M., Silva, L. A., & Benevenuto, F. (2017). A Measurement Study of Hate Speech in Social Media. *In Proceedings of the 28th ACM Conference on Hypertext and Social Media.* Association for Computing Machinery, New York, NY, USA, pp. 85–94.

Morales, E. (2012). Parental Messages Concerning Latino/Black Interracial Dating: An Exploratory Study among Latina/o Young Adults. *Latino Studies*, 10, 314–33.

Newport, F. (2018). Church Leaders and Declining Religious Service Attendance. *Polling Matters, Gallup.* Available online: https://news.gallup.com/opinion/polling -matters/242015/church-leaders-declining-religious-service-attendance.aspx. [Accessed July 20, 2020].

Nilson, S., & Turner, S. E. (2014). *The Colorblind Screen: Television in Post-Racial America.* New York: NYU Press.

O'Neil, N. B. (2007). Socialization of Grandchildren by their Grandparents about the Attitudes and Beliefs of Love and Marriage *OhioLINK Electronic Theses and Dissertations Center*. Retrieved from https://etd.ohiolink.edu/.

Pager, D., & Shepherd, H. (2008). The Sociology of Discrimination: Racial discrimination in employment, housing, credit, and consumer markets. *Annual Review of Sociology,* 34, 181–209.

Parker, J. D., & Madans, J. H. (2002). The Correspondence Between Interracial Births and Multiple-Race Reporting. *American Journal of Public Health,* 92(12), 1976–81.

Parker, K., Morin, R., Horowitz, J. M., & Lopez, M. H. (2015). Multiracial in America: Proud, Diverse and Growing in Numbers. *Pew Research Center's Social & Demographic Trends Project.* Available online: https://www.pewsocialtrends.org /2015/06/11/multiracial-in-america/. [Accessed June 16, 2020].

Parker, K., Anderson, M., & Horowitz, J. M. (2020). Majorities Across Racial, Ethnic Groups Express Support for The Black Lives Matter Movement. *Pew Research Center's Social & Demographic Trends Project.* Available online: https://www .pewsocialtrends.org/2020/06/12/amid-protests-majorities-across-racial-and-ethnic -groups-express-support-for-the-black-lives-matter-movement/ [Accessed June 15, 2020].

Passel, J., Wang, W., & Taylor, P. (2010, June 4). Marrying Out: One-in-Seven New U.S. Marriages Is Interracial or Interethnic. *Pew Research Center's Social & Demographic Trends Project.* https://www.pewresearch.org/social-trends/2010/06 /04/marrying-out/.

Pew Research Center. (2016). On Views of Race and Inequality, Blacks and Whites are Worlds Apart: 1. Demographic Trends and Economic Wellbeing. *Pew Research Center's Social & Demographic Trends Projec*t. Available online: https://www .pewsocialtrends.org/2016/06/27/1-demographic-trends-and-economic-well-being /. [Accessed June 16, 2020].

Polson, E., & Dougherty, K. D. (2019). Worshiping Across the Color Line: The Influence of Congregational Composition on Whites' Friendship Networks and Racial Attitudes. *Sociology of Race and Ethnicity*, 5(1), 100–14.

Quick, K., & Kahlenberg, R. (2019). Attacking the Black–White Opportunity Gap That Comes from Residential Segregation," *The Century Foundation.* Available online: https://tcf.org/content/report/attacking-black-white-opportunity-gap-comes -residential-segregation/. [Accessed 8 May 2020].

Radford, J., & Noe-Bustamante, L. (2019). Immigrants in America: Key Charts and Facts. *Pew Research Center's Hispanic Trends Project.* Available online: https:// www.pewresearch.org/hispanic/2019/06/03/facts-on-u-s-immigrants/. [Accessed June 15, 2020].

Raine, L., & Perrin, A. (2019). Key Findings About Americans' Declining Trust in Government And Each Other *Pew Research Center.* Available online: https://www .pewresearch.org/fact-tank/2019/07/22/key-findings-about-americans-declining -trust-in-government-and-each-other/. [Accessed June 14, 2020].

Roberto, K. A., & Stroes, J. (1992). Grandchildren and Grandparents: Roles, Influences, and Relationships. *The International Journal of Aging and Human Development,* 34(3), 227–39.

Roda, A., & Wells, A. S. (2013). School Choice Policies and Racial Segregation: Where White Parents' Good Intentions, Anxiety, and Privilege Collide. *American Journal of Education,* 119(2), 261–93.

Roth, W. D. (2005). The End of the One-Drop Rule? Labeling of Multiracial Children in Black Intermarriages. *Sociological Forum,* 20, 35–67.

Sears, D., & Savalei, V. (2006). The Political Color Line in America: Many "Peoples of Color" or Black Exceptionalism? *Political Psychology*, 27(6), 895–924.

Shih, M., Wilton, L. S., Does, S., Goodale, B. M., & Sanchez, D. T. (2019). Multiple Racial Identities as Sources of Psychological Resilience." *Social and Personality Psychology Compass*, 13, 1–13.

Thomas, R. J. (2020). Online Exogamy Reconsidered: Estimating the Internet's Effects on Racial, Educational, Religious, Political and Age Assortative Mating. *Social Forces*, 98(3), 1257–86.

Tillman, K., & Miller, B. (2017). The role of family relationships in the psychological wellbeing of interracially dating adolescents. *Social Science Research, 65*, 240–52.

Tillman, K. H., Erichsen, K., Buggs, S. Ga., & Miller, B. New Experiences vs. Old Racism: Intimate Racework and Experiences in Interracial Relationships. Unpublished working paper.

Turner, R. J. (201–). Understanding Health Disparities: The Relevance of the Stress Process Model." *Society & Mental Health,* 3(3), 170–86

Van der Walt, A., & Basson, P. (2015). The Lived Experience of Discrimination of White Women in Committed Interracial Relationships with Black Men" *Indo-Pacific Journal of Phenomenology*, 15(2), 1–16.

Vaquera, E., & Kao, G. (2005). Private and Public Displays of Affection among Interracial and Intra-racial Adolescent Couples." *Social Science Quarterly*, 86(2), 484–509.

Wang, H., Kao, G., & Joyner, K. (2006). Stability of interracial and intraracial romantic relationships among adolescents. *Social Science Research, 35*, 435–53.

Wilton, L. S., Sanchez, D. T., & Garcia, J. (2013). The Stigma of Privilege: Racial Identity and Stigma Consciousness Among Biracial Individuals. *Race and Social Problems*, 5, 41–56.

Wolfe, B. (2015). Racial Integrity Laws (1924–1930)." *Encyclopedia Virginia*. Available online: https://www.encyclopediavirginia.org/Racial_Integrity_Laws_of _the_1920s. [Accessed June 15, 2020].

Yu, Y., & Zhang, Z. (2017). Interracial Marriage and Self-Reported Health of Whites and Blacks in the United States. Population Research and Policy Review, 36(6), 851–70.

Zeigler-Hill, V., Wallace, M. T., & Myers, E. M. (2012). Racial Differences in Self-esteem Revisited: The Role of Impression Management in the Black Self-esteem Advantage *Personality and Individual Differences*, 53, 785–89.

Index

About the Author

Byron Miller, PhD and M.A.T., is associate professor of sociology at the University of South Florida and coordinator for the Interdisciplinary Social Science (ISS) Program. He received a Ph.D. in sociology with a focus on mental health and minor concentration in social stratification from Florida State University, as well as a master's in teaching secondary social science from the University of South Florida. Dr. Miller teaches courses in both sociology and ISS, including Research Methods, Medical Sociology, Sociology of Family, Race and Ethnic Relations, and Introduction to Sociology. His research focuses on racial disparities in health and the impact of interracial romance on health outcomes.

ABOUT THE CONTRIBUTORS

Anthony G. James Jr. is a professor in the Department of Family Science and Social Work at Miami University. His scholar work uses an interdisciplinary approach to understanding social interactions, family science, and human development. He is editor-in-chief of *Marriage & Family Review* and the founder and CEO of Prof_Ajames Enterprises.

Sara Rocks is a sociology PhD student at the University of South Florida studying the sociology of emotions and is passionate about uncovering how emotions shape and are shaped by societal narratives found in confessional media.

Dr. Roudi Nazarinia Roy is associate professor of child development and family studies in the Department of Family and Consumer Sciences at California State University, Long Beach, where she teaches courses on the Transition to Parenthood and Family Dynamics, Family Stress and Coping, and Internships in Child Development and Family Life Education. Her research interests revolve around cultural influences on parental roles across the transition to parenthood and during early childhood, fatherhood engagement, and Multiracial families, as well as the co-author of the book *Biracial Families: Crossing Boundaries, Blending Cultures, and Challenging Racial Ideologies*. Dr. Roy is a certified family life educator through the National Council on Family Relations and serves as a consultant and evaluator for community agencies serving diverse populations of families.

Dr. Kathryn Harker Tillman is professor of sociology at Florida State University, where she currently serves as Chair of the Sociology Department and a research associate within the Center for Demography and Population Health. Dr. Tillman studies the social and health-related outcomes of adolescents and young adults, which a particular focus on the influence of family and interpersonal relationships for individual development, health and risk-taking behaviors, and overall well-being. Current research includes examinations of the social and psychological well-being differences between youth dating same-race and different-race partners, the influence of family structure and relationships upon sexual behavior and romantic relationship formation during the transition to adulthood, the association between youth sexual behavior and psychological and reproductive health outcomes, and the importance of immigrant adaptation for the outcomes of youth and young adults. She received her Ph.D. from the Department of Sociology at the University of North Carolina at Chapel Hill in 2003.

www.ingramcontent.com/pod-product-compliance
Lightning Source LLC
Chambersburg PA
CBHW032353280326
41935CB00008B/555